Baby Boy Names

10,000+ Baby Boy Name Ideas to find the Perfect Name for Your Baby Boy

ISBN: 9798322355038

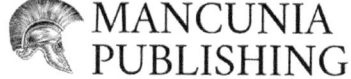

Table of Contents

Introduction..5
Baby Names and Their Origins...7
How to Name Your Baby Boy...10
American baby boy names...13
British baby boy names..16
Canadian baby boy names...19
Australian boy baby names..22
German baby boy names...25
French baby boy names...28
Italian baby boy names...31
Spanish baby boy names...34
Chinese baby boy names..37
Japanese baby boy names..40
Indian baby boy names..43
Mexican baby boy names..46
Brazilian baby boy names..49
Russian baby boy names..52
Dutch baby boy names..55
Swedish baby boy names..58
Norwegian baby boy names..61
Danish baby boy names..64
Finnish baby boy names..67
Greek baby boy names..70
Turkish baby boy names..73
Egyptian baby boy names...76
South African baby boy names...79
Nigerian baby boy names..82
Kenyan baby boy names...85
Ghanaian baby boy names...88
Ethiopian baby boy names..91

Moroccan baby boy names...94
Algerian baby boy names...97
Tunisian baby boy names...100
Libyan baby boy names..103
Saudi Arabian baby boy names..106
Iranian baby boy names..109
Iraqi baby boy names..112
Israeli baby boy names...115
Palestinian baby boy names..118
Jordanian baby boy names..121
Syrian baby boy names..124
Lebanese baby boy names..127
Kuwaiti baby boy names..130
Emirati baby boy names...133
Qatari baby boy names..136
Omani baby boy names...139
Bahraini baby boy names..142
Pakistani baby boy names...145
Bangladeshi baby boy names..148
Sri Lankan baby boy names..151
Nepali baby boy names...154
Bhutanese baby boy names...157
Afghan baby boy names..160
Kazakhstani baby boy names..163
Uzbekistani baby boy names...166
Tajikistani baby boy names...169
Kyrgyzstani baby boy names...172
Turkmenistani baby boy names....................................175
Mongolian baby boy names...178
Vietnamese baby boy names..181
Thai baby boy names...184
Malaysian baby boy names..187
Indonesian baby boy names..190

Filipino baby boy names..193
Singaporean baby boy names...196
Laotian baby boy names..199
Bruneian baby boy names... 202
Taiwanese baby boy names..205
Hong Kong baby boy names..208
Macau baby boy names..211
Tibetan baby boy names... 214
Maldivian baby boy names..217
Mauritian baby boy names...220
Seychellois baby boy names..223
Ancient English Baby Boy Names..226
Royal Baby Boy Names.. 228
Literary Baby Boy Names... 230
Native American Baby Boy Names..234
Aboriginal Baby Boy Names...236
Maroi Baby Boy Names..241
Sami Baby Boy Names... 243
Inuit Baby Boy Names... 245
Hawiian Baby Boy Names...247
Slavic Baby Boy Names... 249
Saxon Baby Boy Names... 251
Nature Based Baby Boy Names... 253
Ancient Irish Baby Boy Names..259

Introduction

Congratulations! The journey of parenthood begins with anticipation, excitement, and perhaps a touch of nervousness. As you prepare to welcome your bundle of joy into the world, one of the most delightful and significant decisions you'll make is choosing the perfect name for your baby boy.

In this book we embark on a heartwarming exploration of the wonderful world of baby names. From timeless classics to modern trends, from cultural treasures to unique gems, this book is your trusted companion on the quest to find the ideal name that will capture the essence of your son and accompany him throughout his life's journey.

With thousands of options to consider, selecting the right name can feel like a daunting task. But fear not! Within these pages, you'll discover a wealth of inspiration, guidance, and practical advice to help you navigate this joyful endeavor with confidence and joy.

Whether you're seeking a name that honors family traditions, reflects your cultural heritage, or simply resonates with your personal style, "Baby Boy Names" offers a diverse array of options to suit every taste and preference. From strong and noble monikers to gentle and poetic choices, there's a name waiting to be discovered that will perfectly complement your precious little one.

But this book is more than just a list of names; it's a celebration of the profound significance of naming and the deep connection it fosters between parent and child. As you peruse these pages, you'll uncover the stories behind the names, the meanings they carry, and the legacies they evoke, inviting you to reflect on the hopes, dreams, and aspirations you hold for your son.

So, whether you're eagerly anticipating the arrival of your baby boy or simply curious about the rich tapestry of names that adorn our world, "Baby Boy Names" is here to inspire, inform, and delight. Let the journey begin as you embark on the enchanting quest to find the perfect name for your little one—a name that will be cherished and loved for a lifetime.

Baby Names and Their Origins

In the wondrous realm of baby names, each moniker carries with it a rich tapestry of history, culture, and meaning. From the familiar to the exotic, the origins of names offer fascinating insights into the diverse traditions and influences that shape our world. In this chapter, we embark on a captivating journey through the origins of baby names, uncovering the stories, symbolism, and significance behind some of the most beloved names for little ones.

Exploring Cultural Heritage -

Names are often deeply rooted in cultural traditions, reflecting the unique identities and histories of different communities around the globe. Whether it's the timeless elegance of European classics like Alexander and Sophia, the rhythmic beauty of African names like Kwame and Aisha, or the lyrical charm of Asian names like Hiroshi and Mei, each culture brings its own distinct flavor to the world of baby names. We'll delve into the origins of these names, tracing their linguistic roots and uncovering the customs and beliefs that have shaped them over centuries.

Meanings and Symbolism -

Beyond their aesthetic appeal, names are imbued with layers of meaning and symbolism that resonate deeply with parents and children alike. From names that evoke strength and courage, like Ethan and Valentina, to those that embody beauty and grace, like Adonis and Isabella, the meanings behind names can often reflect the hopes, aspirations, and values of parents.

Influence of Literature and Mythology -

Throughout history, literature and mythology have served as wellsprings of inspiration for baby names, offering a treasure trove of timeless classics and legendary figures to draw upon. From the heroic exploits of Arthurian legends, which give rise to names like Arthur and Guinevere, to the mystical allure of Greek mythology, which inspires names like Apollo and Athena, the world of storytelling is brimming with names that capture the imagination and stir the soul. We'll delve into the stories behind these iconic names, exploring the enduring appeal of literary and mythological figures as sources of inspiration for parents seeking names that are both timeless and evocative.

Trends and Innovations -

As society evolves and cultures intersect, the landscape of baby names is constantly evolving, giving rise to new trends and innovations in naming practices. From the rise of gender-neutral names like Taylor and Jordan to the resurgence of vintage names like Eleanor and Theodore, we'll explore the latest trends shaping the world of baby names and the cultural forces driving these shifts. We'll also examine the growing influence of pop culture, technology, and celebrity culture on naming trends, highlighting the ways in which modern parents are redefining the boundaries of traditional naming conventions.

Embracing Diversity and Inclusivity -

In an increasingly interconnected world, diversity and inclusivity have become guiding principles in the realm of baby names, reflecting a growing recognition of the rich tapestry of human experience. We'll celebrate the diversity of names from around the world, highlighting the importance of embracing cultural diversity and honoring the unique identities of every child. From multicultural names that bridge linguistic and cultural divides to names that celebrate ethnic heritage and LGBTQ+ identities, we'll explore the ways in which naming practices are evolving to reflect the inclusive values of modern society.

How to Name Your Baby Boy...

Naming your baby boy is one of the most joyous and meaningful tasks you'll undertake as a parent. From navigating the endless array of options to ensuring that the chosen name reflects your values and aspirations, the process of finding the perfect name can be both exhilarating and overwhelming. In this chapter, we'll guide you through the steps to naming your baby boy with confidence and clarity.

1. Start Early and Do Your Research -
Naming your baby is a decision that deserves careful consideration, so it's never too early to start brainstorming ideas. Begin by exploring a variety of sources for inspiration, from baby name books and websites to family traditions and cultural heritage. Keep a running list of names that catch your eye, and don't be afraid to think outside the box.

2. Consider Your Values and Aspirations -
As you narrow down your list of potential names, take some time to reflect on the values and aspirations you hope to instill in your son. Consider the meanings and symbolism associated with each name, as well as how it aligns with your family's cultural heritage and personal beliefs. Whether you're drawn to names that evoke strength and resilience or those that celebrate creativity and compassion, choose a name that resonates with the vision you have for your child's future.

3. Think About Sound and Flow -
The sound and rhythm of a name can have a significant impact on its overall appeal and how it will be perceived by others. Pay attention to the way each name sounds when spoken aloud, as well as how it pairs with your last name. Avoid names that are difficult to pronounce or spell, and

consider how the name will sound in different contexts, from the playground to the boardroom.

4. Get Feedback from Loved Ones -
Once you've narrowed down your list to a few favorite names, don't hesitate to seek feedback from trusted friends and family members. They may offer valuable insights and perspectives that can help you make your final decision. Keep in mind, however, that ultimately the decision is yours and your partner's, so trust your instincts and choose a name that feels right to you.

5. Consider the Long Term -
While it's important to choose a name that you love in the moment, it's also crucial to consider how the name will age with your child. Think about how the name will sound at different stages of life, from infancy to adulthood, and whether it will still feel appropriate and relevant in the years to come. Avoid trendy or overly unique names that may feel dated or out of place as your child grows older.

6. Embrace Your Creativity -
Don't be afraid to think outside the box and explore unconventional or unexpected names that speak to your unique sense of style and personality. Whether you're drawn to literary references, nature-inspired names, or quirky pop culture references, embrace your creativity and choose a name that reflects the one-of-a-kind spirit of your little one.

7. Trust Your Instincts -
At the end of the day, the most important thing is to choose a name that feels right to you and your partner. Trust your instincts and listen to your heart as you make this deeply personal decision.

American baby boy names

1. Aaron - Exalted, strong
2. Alexander - Defender of men
3. Andrew - Manly, brave
4. Anthony - Priceless
5. Benjamin - Son of the right hand
6. Brandon - From the broom hill
7. Caleb - Faithful, bold
8. Daniel - God is my judge
9. David - Beloved
10. Ethan - Firm, enduring
11. Frank - Free man
12. George - Farmer
13. Henry - Ruler of the home
14. Isaac - He will laugh
15. Jacob - Supplanter
16. James - Supplanter
17. John - God is gracious
18. Joseph - He will add
19. Joshua - God is salvation
20. Justin - Just, fair
21. Kevin - Kind, gentle
22. Liam - Strong-willed warrior
23. Luke - Light giving
24. Matthew - Gift of God
25. Michael - Who is like God?
26. Nathan - He gave
27. Nicholas - Victory of the people
28. Oliver - Olive tree
29. Patrick - Nobleman
30. Peter - Rock
31. Robert - Bright fame
32. Samuel - God has heard
33. Thomas - Twin

34. William - Resolute protector
35. Zachary - The Lord has remembered
36. Adam - Man, to make
37. Brian - High, noble
38. Charles - Free man
39. Derek - Ruler of the people
40. Edward - Wealthy guardian
41. Fred - Peaceful ruler
42. Gregory - Watchful, alert
43. Harry - Army ruler
44. Ian - God is gracious
45. Jesse - Gift
46. Kyle - Narrow
47. Lewis - Renowned warrior
48. Mark - Warlike
49. Neil - Champion
50. Owen - Young warrior
51. Paul - Humble
52. Quentin - Fifth
53. Richard - Brave ruler
54. Steven - Crown
55. Timothy - Honoring God
56. Vincent - Conquering
57. Walter - Army ruler
58. Xavier - New house
59. Yale - Heights, upland
60. Zane - God is gracious
61. Albert - Noble, bright
62. Bruce - From the brushwood thicket
63. Carl - Free man
64. Dean - Valley
65. Ernest - Serious, determined
66. Felix - Happy, fortunate
67. Glenn - Valley
68. Howard - High guardian
69. Ivan - God is gracious

70. Jerome - Sacred name
71. Kent - High or coastal land
72. Leonard - Brave lion
73. Morris - Dark-skinned
74. Norman - Northman
75. Orville - Gold town
76. Philip - Lover of horses
77. Ralph - Wolf counsel
78. Stanley - Near the stony clearing
79. Troy - Foot soldier
80. Vernon - Alder tree
81. Wayne - Wagon maker
82. Arnold - Eagle power
83. Barry - Fair-headed
84. Clifford - Ford near a slope
85. Dennis - God of wine
86. Edgar - Wealthy spearman
87. Floyd - Gray-haired
88. Gerald - Ruler with the spear
89. Horace - Timekeeper
90. Irving - Green river
91. Jonah - Dove
92. Kirk - Church
93. Lionel - Lion
94. Monroe - Mouth of the Roe river
95. Nigel - Champion
96. Oscar - Friend of deer
97. Preston - Priest's town
98. Rupert - Bright fame
99. Sheldon - Steep valley
100. Tyson - Firebrand

British baby boy names

1. Aaron - High mountain, exalted
2. Adam - Man, to make
3. Adrian - Dark one
4. Alfred - Wise counselor
5. Alexander - Defender of mankind
6. Andrew - Manly, brave
7. Anthony - Priceless one
8. Arthur - Bear, strong
9. Benjamin - Son of the right hand
10. Blake - Fair-haired, dark
11. Bradley - Broad clearing
12. Brandon - Broom hill
13. Brian - High, noble
14. Charles - Free man
15. Christopher - Christ-bearer
16. Colin - Young creature
17. Daniel - God is my judge
18. David - Beloved
19. Dominic - Lordly, belonging to God
20. Edward - Wealthy guardian
21. Ethan - Firm, strong
22. Felix - Happy, fortunate
23. George - Farmer
24. Graham - Gravelly homestead
25. Harry - Army ruler
26. Henry - Ruler of the home
27. Ian - God is gracious
28. Isaac - Laughter
29. Jack - God is gracious
30. James - Supplanter
31. Jason - Healer
32. Jonathan - God has given
33. Joseph - God will increase

34. Joshua - The Lord is my salvation
35. Justin - Just, fair
36. Keith - Wood
37. Kenneth - Handsome
38. Kevin - Kind, gentle, handsome
39. Lawrence - From Laurentum
40. Lewis - Renowned warrior
41. Liam - Will, desire, helmet, protection
42. Luke - Light giving
43. Martin - Warlike
44. Matthew - Gift of God
45. Michael - Who is like God?
46. Nathan - He gave
47. Neil - Champion
48. Oliver - Olive tree
49. Owen - Young warrior
50. Patrick - Nobleman
51. Paul - Small, humble
52. Peter - Rock
53. Philip - Lover of horses
54. Ralph - Wolf counsel
55. Richard - Brave ruler
56. Robert - Bright fame
57. Roger - Famous spear
58. Ronald - Ruler's counselor
59. Samuel - God has heard
60. Sean - God is gracious
61. Simon - He has heard
62. Stephen - Crown, garland
63. Thomas - Twin
64. Timothy - Honoring God
65. Toby - God is good
66. Trevor - Large settlement
67. Vincent - Conquering
68. William - Resolute protection
69. Zachary - The Lord has remembered

70. Albert - Noble, bright
71. Benedict - Blessed
72. Caleb - Faithful, bold
73. Derek - Ruler of the people
74. Elijah - The Lord is my God
75. Frederick - Peaceful ruler
76. Gabriel - God is my strength
77. Hugo - Mind, intellect
78. Isaiah - Salvation of the Lord
79. Jasper - Treasurer
80. Leonard - Brave as a lion
81. Maximilian - Greatest
82. Noah - Rest, comfort
83. Oscar - God spear, deer-lover
84. Quentin - Fifth
85. Rupert - Bright fame
86. Stanley - Near the stony clearing
87. Theodore - God-given
88. Victor - Conqueror
89. Walter - Army ruler
90. Xavier - New house
91. Arnold - Eagle power
92. Basil - Royal, kingly
93. Clifford - Ford by a cliff
94. Desmond - From South Munster
95. Edgar - Wealthy spear-man
96. Franklin - Free landholder
97. Gerald - Ruler with the spear
98. Howard - High guardian
99. Ivan - God is gracious
100. Leonard - Lion strength

Canadian baby boy names

1. Aaron - High mountain
2. Adam - Man
3. Adrian - From Hadria
4. Aidan - Little fiery one
5. Alexander - Defender of mankind
6. Andrew - Manly
7. Anthony - Priceless
8. Austin - Majestic
9. Benjamin - Son of the right hand
10. Blake - Pale blond one
11. Brandon - From the broom hill
12. Caleb - Whole hearted
13. Cameron - Crooked nose
14. Charles - Free man
15. Christopher - Christ-bearer
16. Connor - Lover of hounds
17. Daniel - God is my judge
18. David - Beloved
19. Dylan - Son of the sea
20. Ethan - Firm, enduring
21. Evan - God is gracious
22. Felix - Happy, fortunate
23. Gabriel - God is my strength
24. George - Farmer
25. Henry - Estate ruler
26. Isaac - He will laugh
27. Jack - God is gracious
28. Jacob - Supplanter
29. James - Supplanter
30. Jason - Healer
31. Jonathan - God has given
32. Joseph - He will add
33. Joshua - The Lord is my salvation

34. Justin - Just, fair
35. Keith - Wood
36. Kevin - Gentle birth
37. Kyle - Narrow
38. Liam - Strong-willed warrior
39. Lucas - Light
40. Luke - Light
41. Mark - Warlike
42. Matthew - Gift of God
43. Michael - Who is like God?
44. Nathan - He gave
45. Nicholas - Victory of the people
46. Noah - Rest, comfort
47. Oliver - Olive tree
48. Owen - Young warrior
49. Patrick - Nobleman
50. Paul - Small
51. Peter - Rock
52. Philip - Lover of horses
53. Richard - Brave power
54. Robert - Bright fame
55. Ryan - Little king
56. Samuel - God has heard
57. Sean - God is gracious
58. Sebastian - Venerable
59. Simon - He has heard
60. Stephen - Crown
61. Thomas - Twin
62. Timothy - Honoring God
63. William - Resolute protector
64. Xavier - New house
65. Zachary - The Lord has remembered
66. Aaron - High mountain
67. Bennett - Little blessed one
68. Carson - Son of the marsh-dwellers
69. Dominic - Belonging to God

70. Eli - Ascended
71. Finn - Fair
72. Graham - Gravelly homestead
73. Harrison - Son of Harry
74. Ian - God is gracious
75. Jared - He descends
76. Kaden - Companion
77. Levi - Joined, attached
78. Maddox - Son of Madoc
79. Nolan - Champion
80. Orion - Rising in the sky
81. Preston - Priest's town
82. Quentin - Fifth
83. Riley - Rye clearing
84. Sawyer - Woodcutter
85. Tristan - Tumult
86. Uriah - God is my light
87. Vincent - Conquering
88. Wyatt - Brave in war
89. Xander - Defender of the people
90. Yale - Fertile upland
91. Zane - God is gracious
92. Abel - Breath
93. Baxter - Baker
94. Cedric - Bounty
95. Drake - Dragon
96. Emery - Industrious
97. Fletcher - Arrow-maker
98. Gunner - Bold warrior
99. Hugo - Mind, intellect
100. Ivan - God is gracious

Australian boy baby names

1. Aaron – High mountain
2. Aidan – Little fiery one
3. Alexander – Defender of men
4. Angus – One strength
5. Ashton – Ash tree town
6. Bailey – Law enforcer
7. Benjamin – Son of the right hand
8. Blake – Pale blond one or dark
9. Bradley – Broad clearing
10. Brandon – Broom hill
11. Braxton – Brock's town
12. Bryce – Speckled
13. Caleb – Faithful
14. Callum – Dove
15. Cameron – Crooked nose
16. Charlie – Free man
17. Christian – Follower of Christ
18. Connor – Lover of hounds
19. Cooper – Barrel maker
20. Daniel – God is my judge
21. Declan – Man of prayer
22. Dylan – Son of the sea
23. Ethan – Firm, enduring
24. Felix – Happy, fortunate
25. Finley – Fair-haired hero
26. Flynn – Son of the red-haired one
27. Gabriel – God is my strength
28. George – Farmer
29. Harrison – Son of Harry
30. Harvey – Battle worthy
31. Hayden – Fire
32. Henry – Ruler of the home
33. Hugo – Bright in mind and spirit

34. Isaac – He will laugh
35. Jack – God is gracious
36. Jacob – Supplanter
37. James – Supplanter
38. Jasper – Treasurer
39. Jayden – Thankful
40. Jesse – Gift
41. Joel – God is willing
42. John – God is gracious
43. Jordan – Descend or flow down
44. Joshua – The Lord is my salvation
45. Julian – Youthful
46. Kai – Sea
47. Kaiden – Fighter
48. Kian – Ancient
49. Kyle – Narrow strait
50. Lachlan – From the land of lakes
51. Leo – Lion
52. Liam – Resolute protector
53. Lincoln – Town by the pool
54. Logan – Small hollow
55. Lucas – Light-giving
56. Mason – Stone worker
57. Matthew – Gift of God
58. Max – Greatest
59. Michael – Who is like God?
60. Miles – Soldier
61. Mitchell – Who is like God?
62. Nathan – He gave
63. Nathaniel – Gift of God
64. Noah – Rest, comfort
65. Oliver – Olive tree
66. Oscar – Divine spear
67. Owen – Young warrior
68. Patrick – Nobleman
69. Paul – Small

70. Peter – Rock
71. Phoenix – Dark red
72. Reuben – Behold, a son
73. Rhys – Enthusiasm
74. Riley – Rye clearing
75. Ryan – Little king
76. Samuel – God has heard
77. Sebastian – Venerable
78. Seth – Appointed
79. Spencer – Steward
80. Stanley – Near the stony meadow
81. Thomas – Twin
82. Timothy – Honoring God
83. Tristan – Tumult
84. Tyler – Tile maker
85. Victor – Conqueror
86. Vincent – Conquering
87. William – Resolute protector
88. Xavier – The new house
89. Zachary – The Lord has remembered
90. Zane – God is gracious
91. Adam – Man
92. Adrian – Sea or water
93. Aiden – Little and fiery
94. Alfred – Wise counselor
95. Andrew – Manly and strong
96. Anthony – Priceless one
97. Archer – Bowman
98. Austin – Majestic dignity
99. Bentley – Meadow with coarse grass
100. Cody – Helpful

German baby boy names

1. Aaron – Enlightened
2. Adrian – Sea or water
3. Albert – Noble and bright
4. Alexander – Defender of mankind
5. Andreas – Strong and manly
6. Anton – Priceless
7. Benjamin – Son of the right hand
8. Bernd – Brave as a bear
9. Bruno – Brown
10. Carl – Free man
11. Christian – Follower of Christ
12. Christoph – Bearer of Christ
13. Daniel – God is my judge
14. David – Beloved
15. Dieter – Ruler of the people
16. Dominik – Belonging to the Lord
17. Emil – Rival
18. Erik – Ever ruler
19. Fabian – Bean grower
20. Felix – Happy and fortunate
21. Florian – Flowering
22. Franz – Free man
23. Friedrich – Peaceful ruler
24. Georg – Farmer
25. Gerhard – Strong spear
26. Gustav – Staff of the Goths
27. Hans – God is gracious
28. Heinrich – Ruler of the household
29. Hermann – Army man
30. Horst – Man from the forest
31. Jakob – Supplanter
32. Jens – God is gracious
33. Johann – God is gracious

34. Jonas – Dove
35. Jürgen – Earth worker
36. Karl – Free man
37. Klaus – Victory of the people
38. Konrad – Brave counsel
39. Lars – Crowned with laurel
40. Leon – Lion
41. Lorenz – From Laurentum
42. Lucas – Light
43. Ludwig – Famous warrior
44. Lukas – Light
45. Manuel – God is with us
46. Marcel – Little warrior
47. Markus – Warlike
48. Martin – Warlike
49. Matthias – Gift of God
50. Max – The greatest
51. Michael – Who is like God?
52. Moritz – Dark-skinned
53. Nico – Victory of the people
54. Oliver – Olive tree
55. Oscar – God's spear
56. Paul – Small
57. Peter – Rock
58. Phillip – Lover of horses
59. Rainer – Deciding warrior
60. Reinhard – Strong counsel
61. Robert – Bright fame
62. Rolf – Famous wolf
63. Sebastian – Venerable
64. Simon – He who hears
65. Stefan – Crown
66. Thomas – Twin
67. Tim – Honoring God
68. Tobias – God is good
69. Uwe – Inheritance

70. Valentin – Strong, healthy
71. Viktor – Conqueror
72. Vincent – Conquering
73. Werner – Defending army
74. Wilhelm – Determined protector
75. Wolfgang – Wolf journey
76. Xavier – New house
77. Yannick – God is gracious
78. Zacharias – God has remembered
79. Armin – Whole, universal
80. Bastian – Venerable
81. Caspar – Treasurer
82. Claus – Victory of the people
83. Detlef – Heritage of the people
84. Eberhard – Strong as a boar
85. Fritz – Peaceful ruler
86. Gotthard – God-hard
87. Harald – Leader of the army
88. Ingmar – Famous son
89. Joachim – God will establish
90. Leopold – Bold people
91. Norbert – Bright north
92. Otmar – Famous wealth
93. Rüdiger – Famous spear
94. Siegfried – Victorious peace
95. Theodor – Gift of God
96. Ulrich – Powerful and prosperous
97. Volker – People's guard
98. Waldemar – Famous ruler
99. Xaver – New house
100. York – Boar estate

French baby boy names

1. Adrien – Dark one
2. Alexandre – Defender of mankind
3. Alain – Harmony, stone, or noble
4. Antoine – Priceless one
5. Armand – Soldier
6. Andre – Manly, brave
7. Baptiste – Baptist
8. Benoit – Blessed
9. Bernard – Brave as a bear
10. Blaise – Lisp, stutter
11. Bruno – Brown
12. Charles – Free man
13. Christophe – Christ-bearer
14. Claude – Lame, crippled
15. Damien – To tame
16. Daniel – God is my judge
17. David – Beloved
18. Denis – God of wine
19. Dominique – Of the Lord
20. Edouard – Wealthy guardian
21. Emile – Industrious
22. Eric – Eternal ruler
23. Fabien – Bean grower
24. Felix – Happy, fortunate
25. Francis – Free man
26. Frederic – Peaceful ruler
27. Gabriel – God is my strength
28. Gaston – Guest, stranger
29. Gerard – Strong like a spear
30. Gilles – Shield of goatskin
31. Guillaume – Resolute protector
32. Henri – Ruler of the home
33. Hugo – Mind, intellect

34. Isaac – He will laugh
35. Jacques – Supplanter
36. Jean – God is gracious
37. Jerome – Sacred name
38. Joel – Jehovah is God
39. Julien – Youthful, downy
40. Laurent – From Laurentum, Italy
41. Louis – Famous warrior
42. Luc – Light
43. Marcel – Little warrior
44. Mathieu – Gift of God
45. Maxime – Greatest
46. Michel – Who is like God?
47. Nicolas – Victory of the people
48. Olivier – Olive tree
49. Pascal – Born on Passover
50. Patrice – Nobleman
51. Paul – Small
52. Philippe – Lover of horses
53. Pierre – Rock
54. Quentin – Fifth
55. Raphael – God has healed
56. Raoul – Wolf counsel
57. Raymond – Wise protector
58. Renaud – Wise power
59. Richard – Brave ruler
60. Robert – Bright fame
61. Roger – Famous spear
62. Roland – Famous land
63. Romain – From Rome
64. Sebastien – Venerable, revered
65. Serge – Servant
66. Simon – He who hears
67. Stephane – Crown
68. Sylvain – Of the forest
69. Theodore – Gift of God

70. Thierry – Ruler of the people
71. Thomas – Twin
72. Valentin – Strong, healthy
73. Vincent – Conquering
74. Yves – Yew wood
75. Zacharie – God remembers
76. Abel – Breath
77. Achille – Pain
78. Adolphe – Noble wolf
79. Amaury – Work power
80. Anatole – From the east
81. Auguste – Great, magnificent
82. Barthelemy – Son of Talmai (farmer)
83. Basile – Kingly
84. Celestin – Heavenly
85. Clement – Merciful
86. Cyrille – Lordly, masterful
87. Desire – Desired
88. Elie – My God is Yahweh
89. Eloi – Chosen
90. Etienne – Crown
91. Evrard – Strong boar
92. Fergus – Man of force
93. Gregoire – Watchful, alert
94. Herve – Battle glory
95. Ignace – Fiery one
96. Jules – Youthful
97. Leon – Lion
98. Maurice – Dark-skinned
99. Noe – Rest, comfort
100. Odilon – Wealthy, fortunate

Italian baby boy names

1. Alessandro – Defender of mankind
2. Alberto – Noble and bright
3. Antonio – Priceless one
4. Adriano – Dark one
5. Angelo – Messenger of God
6. Arturo – Bear
7. Benito – Blessed
8. Carlo – Free man
9. Cesare – Long haired
10. Dante – Enduring
11. Dario – Possess
12. Elio – Sun
13. Enzo – Ruler of the household
14. Fabio – Bean grower
15. Federico – Peaceful ruler
16. Gianni – God is gracious
17. Giulio – Youthful
18. Giovanni – God is gracious
19. Giuseppe – He will add
20. Ignazio – Fiery
21. Leonardo – Brave as a lion
22. Lorenzo – Man from Laurentum
23. Luca – Light
24. Marco – Warlike
25. Mario – Bitter
26. Matteo – Gift of God
27. Mauro – Dark skinned
28. Nicolo – Victory of the people
29. Orlando – Famous land
30. Pietro – Rock
31. Riccardo – Brave ruler
32. Roberto – Bright fame
33. Sergio – Servant

34. Stefano – Crown
35. Tommaso – Twin
36. Umberto – Bright bear
37. Valentino – Strong, healthy
38. Vincenzo – Conquering
39. Alessio – Defender
40. Anselmo – Divine protection
41. Bartolomeo – Son of Talmai
42. Biagio – Stammering
43. Bruno – Brown
44. Claudio – Lame
45. Corrado – Bold counselor
46. Diego – Supplanter
47. Edoardo – Wealthy guardian
48. Emilio – Rival
49. Eugenio – Well-born
50. Fabrizio – Craftsman
51. Filippo – Friend of horses
52. Franco – Frenchman
53. Gerardo – Spear rule
54. Guglielmo – Will helmet
55. Iacopo – Supplanter
56. Isidoro – Gift of Isis
57. Lazzaro – God has helped
58. Leandro – Lion man
59. Ludovico – Famous warrior
60. Massimo – Greatest
61. Nazario – From Nazareth
62. Osvaldo – God's power
63. Paolo – Small
64. Quintino – Fifth
65. Raffaele – God has healed
66. Renato – Reborn
67. Rocco – Rest
68. Salvatore – Savior
69. Tiziano – Giant

70. Ugo – Mind, heart, spirit
71. Vito – Life
72. Zeno – Gift of Zeus
73. Adriano – Dark
74. Alonzo – Noble, ready
75. Amedeo – Love of God
76. Beppe – He will add
77. Ciro – Like the sun
78. Domenico – Belonging to the Lord
79. Emanuele – God is with us
80. Ernesto – Serious, determined
81. Felice – Happy, lucky
82. Gaetano – From Gaeta
83. Gino – Short form of names ending in 'gino'
84. Horatio – Timekeeper
85. Italo – From Italy
86. Lino – A cry of grief
87. Marcello – Little warrior
88. Nino – God is gracious
89. Orazio – Has good eyesight
90. Pasquale – Related to Easter
91. Quirino – Spear
92. Rosario – Rosary
93. Silvio – Wood, forest
94. Teodoro – Gift of God
95. Ubaldo – Bold and brave
96. Valentino – Healthy, strong
97. Virgilio – Staff bearer
98. Yago – Supplanter
99. Zan – God is gracious
100. Alessio – Defender

Spanish baby boy names

1. Alejandro – Defender of mankind
2. Antonio – Priceless one
3. Carlos – Free man
4. Diego – Supplanter
5. Eduardo – Wealthy guardian
6. Felipe – Lover of horses
7. Gabriel – God is my strength
8. Hugo – Mind, intellect
9. Ignacio – Fiery one
10. Javier – Bright
11. Lorenzo – From Laurentum
12. Manuel – God is with us
13. Nicolas – Victory of the people
14. Oscar – Divine spear
15. Pablo – Small
16. Rafael – God has healed
17. Sergio – Servant
18. Tomas – Twin
19. Vicente – Conquering
20. Francisco – Free man
21. Andres – Manly, brave
22. Fernando – Adventurous, bold journey
23. Juan – God is gracious
24. Mario – Sailor
25. Pedro – Rock
26. Roberto – Bright fame
27. Santiago – Saint James
28. Victor – Conqueror
29. Miguel – Who is like God?
30. Jose – God will increase
31. Enrique – Ruler of the home
32. Jesus – God rescues
33. Alberto – Noble, bright

34. Arturo – Bear
35. Daniel – God is my judge
36. David – Beloved
37. Esteban – Crown
38. Guillermo – Resolute protector
39. Luis – Famous warrior
40. Marcos – Warlike
41. Ramon – Wise protector
42. Ricardo – Powerful ruler
43. Rodrigo – Famous ruler
44. Angel – Messenger of God
45. Armando – Soldier
46. Benito – Blessed
47. Cristian – Follower of Christ
48. Ernesto – Serious, resolute
49. Gerardo – Spear rule
50. Julio – Youthful
51. Leonardo – Brave lion
52. Martin – Warlike
53. Maximiliano – Greatest
54. Ruben – Behold, a son
55. Salvador – Savior
56. Alfonso – Noble, ready
57. Bruno – Brown
58. Emilio – Rival
59. Gregorio – Watchful, alert
60. Joaquin – God will establish
61. Mateo – Gift of God
62. Patricio – Nobleman
63. Raul – Wolf counsel
64. Samuel – God has heard
65. Teodoro – Gift of God
66. Adan – Man, earth
67. Cesar – Long-haired
68. Domingo – Lord's child
69. Fabian – Bean grower

70. Ismael – God will hear
71. Marcelo – Little warrior
72. Octavio – Eighth
73. Pascual – Born on Passover
74. Saul – Asked for, prayed for
75. Valentino – Brave, strong
76. Alfredo – Elf counsel
77. Bernardo – Brave as a bear
78. Ezequiel – God will strengthen
79. Horacio – Timekeeper
80. Luciano – Light
81. Narciso – Sleep, numbness
82. Orlando – Famous land
83. Placido – Calm, quiet
84. Rolando – Famous throughout the land
85. Silvio – Wood, forest
86. Abelardo – Noble, resolute
87. Amadeo – Love of God
88. Claudio – Lame
89. Dionisio – God of wine
90. Humberto – Bright warrior
91. Jacinto – Hyacinth
92. Leandro – Lion man
93. Norberto – Bright north
94. Quinton – Fifth
95. Romulo – Citizen of Rome
96. Timoteo – Honoring God
97. Ulises – Wrathful
98. Virgilio – Staff bearer
99. Zacarias – God remembers
100. Isidro – Gift of Isis

Chinese baby boy names

1. Li – Strong
2. Wang – King
3. Zhang – Archer
4. Liu – Kill, destroy
5. Chen – Great
6. Yang – Poplar
7. Huang – Yellow
8. Zhao – Enlightened
9. Wu – Military
10. Zhou – State
11. Xu – Slow
12. Sun – Descendant
13. Ma – Horse
14. Zhu – Vermilion
15. Hu – Tiger
16. Guo – Country
17. He – River
18. Lin – Forest
19. Gao – High
20. Luo – Camel
21. Zheng – Government
22. Liang – Bright
23. Feng – Maple
24. Song – Pine tree
25. Dong – East
26. Han – Korean
27. Tao – Peach
28. Jiang – River
29. Qi – Enlighten
30. Yuan – Original
31. Zeng – Increase
32. Peng – Roc bird
33. Tang – Chinese dynasty

34. Yin – Silver
35. Long – Dragon
36. Lei – Thunder
37. Zhou – Continent
38. Zou – Walk slowly
39. Shi – Lion
40. Cui – Green
41. Du – Capital
42. Yu – Universe
43. Su – Plain
44. Ye – Leaf
45. Lu – Deer
46. Zhang – Long
47. Wei – Power
48. Xu – Sunrise
49. Xie – Thank
50. Qian – Money
51. Shen – Deep
52. Zhu – Bamboo
53. Fan – Ordinary
54. Rong – Glory
55. Guan – Mountain pass
56. Zhan – Spread out
57. Fu – Wealthy
58. Qu – Song
59. Shao – Young
60. Yu – Rain
61. Hao – Good
62. Bian – Flat
63. Xiong – Bear
64. Yuan – Destiny
65. Jing – Quiet
66. Yue – Moon
67. Cao – Grass
68. Ding – Top
69. Tian – Field

70. Zuo – Left
71. Bao – Treasure
72. Ji – Lucky
73. Liao – Distant
74. Qiu – Autumn
75. Yan – Swallow bird
76. Fei – Fly
77. Mao – Fur
78. Pan – Plate
79. Bao – Leopard
80. Shu – Kind
81. Zang – Hide
82. Chai – Firewood
83. Du – Stomach
84. Qin – Zither
85. Xuan – Mysterious
86. Ning – Peaceful
87. Kan – Look
88. Lan – Orchid
89. Tong – Bronze
90. Jiang – Ginger
91. Rui – Sharp
92. Zhi – Wisdom
93. Wen – Culture
94. Xia – Glow of the sunrise
95. Shun – Smooth
96. Yi – Righteous
97. An – Peace
98. Hui – Kind
99. Jun – Ruler
100. Ming – Bright

Japanese baby boy names

1. Akio – Bright Man
2. Akihiko – Bright Prince
3. Akira – Bright, Clear
4. Asahi – Morning Sun
5. Atsushi – Industrious Director
6. Daiki – Great Radiance
7. Eiji – Eternity Order
8. Fumio – Scholarly Hero
9. Goro – Fifth Son
10. Haruki – Shining Sun
11. Hideo – Excellent Man
12. Hiroshi – Generous
13. Ichiro – First Son
14. Isamu – Courage
15. Jiro – Second Son
16. Junichi – Obedient One
17. Kaito – Ocean Flying
18. Kazuki – Harmonious Hope
19. Kei – Blessing
20. Kenji – Strong and Vigorous
21. Kenta – Large, Strong
22. Kiyoshi – Pure
23. Makoto – Sincerity
24. Masaru – Victory
25. Michio – Man on a Journey
26. Minoru – Truth
27. Naoki – Straight Tree
28. Nobu – Faith
29. Osamu – Disciplined, Studious
30. Riku – Land
31. Ryo – Cool, Refreshing
32. Satoshi – Wise, Fast Learner
33. Shigeru – Luxuriant

34. Shin – True, Genuine
35. Shiro – Fourth Son
36. Susumu – Progress
37. Tadao – Loyal, Faithful Man
38. Takashi – Noble, Prosperous
39. Takeo – Warrior Hero
40. Taro – First Son
41. Tomo – Knowledge, Wisdom
42. Toru – Persistent, Clear
43. Yasu – Peace
44. Yoshi – Lucky, Righteous
45. Yuji – Courageous Second Son
46. Yuki – Happiness, Snow
47. Yukio – Blessed Hero
48. Yutaka – Abundant
49. Yuuto – Gentle Person
50. Zen – Meditation
51. Hideaki – Excellent Brightness
52. Kichiro – Lucky Son
53. Masaaki – True Brightness
54. Masayuki – Happiness, Blessing
55. Naoto – Honest Person
56. Ryota – Clear, Refreshing
57. Satoru – Enlightenment
58. Seiji – Lawful, Manage
59. Shoji – Correct Second Son
60. Takuma – Open Truth
61. Tetsuya – Philosophy, Clear
62. Tsuyoshi – Strong, Tough
63. Yasushi – Peaceful
64. Yoshito – Righteous Person
65. Yuichi – Kind First Son
66. Yusei – Star
67. Daichi – Great Wisdom
68. Etsu – Delight
69. Hiroto – Large Flying

70. Itsuki – Tree
71. Kaoru – Fragrance
72. Kyo – Cooperation
73. Masato – Correct Person
74. Osamu – Studious
75. Ren – Love, Lotus
76. Ryoichi – Good First Son
77. Sora – Sky
78. Taiga – Great, Big
79. Yori – Trust
80. Yuma – Calm Truth
81. Aoi – Blue, Green
82. Haruto – Sun Flying
83. Koki – Light, Hope
84. Masa – Just, True
85. Naoki – Honest Tree
86. Riku – Land, Continent
87. Shota – Soaring, Large
88. Toshi – Wise, Alert
89. Yu – Gentle
90. Yuto – Tender
91. Akito – Bright Person
92. Hiro – Generous
93. Issey – First Born
94. Kaito – Sea, Ocean
95. Kyo – Cooperation
96. Masa – Just, True
97. Ryo – Cool, Refresh
98. Sota – Sudden, Sound
99. Toshi – Wise, Alert
100. Yuta – Calm

Indian baby boy names

1. Aarav – Peaceful
2. Vivaan – Full of life
3. Aditya – The sun
4. Aryan – Noble
5. Arjun – Bright, shining
6. Atharv – First Veda
7. Shaurya – Bravery
8. Harshit – Joyful
9. Yuvan – Youthful
10. Advait – Unique
11. Siddharth – One who has attained enlightenment
12. Dhruv – Constant, faithful
13. Ishaan – The sun
14. Aarush – First rays of the sun
15. Pranav – Sacred syllable OM
16. Keshav – Another name for Lord Krishna
17. Rudra – Lord Shiva
18. Abhinav – New, young
19. Aadi – Beginning
20. Ayush – Long life
21. Aman – Peace
22. Anirudh – Unstoppable
23. Hrithik – From the heart
24. Lakshya – Aim
25. Om – Sacred syllable in Hinduism
26. Parth – Another name for Arjuna
27. Rishabh – Morality
28. Tanmay – Engrossed
29. Utkarsh – Progress
30. Vedant – Ultimate knowledge
31. Yash – Fame
32. Alok – Light
33. Bhavesh – Lord of the world

34. Chirag – Lamp
35. Daksh – Competent
36. Eklavya – Student who learned bow by watching
37. Farhan – Joyful
38. Girish – Lord of mountains
39. Harman – Everybody's beloved
40. Ishan – Sun
41. Jai – Victory
42. Kunal – Lotus
43. Lokesh – King of the world
44. Manish – God of mind
45. Naman – Salutation
46. Ojas – Vitality
47. Prithvi – Earth
48. Rajat – Silver
49. Surya – Sun
50. Tarun – Young
51. Uday – To rise
52. Varun – Lord of water
53. Yuvraj – Prince
54. Akshay – Immortal
55. Bijoy – Victory
56. Chetan – Consciousness
57. Dhanush – Bow
58. Eeshan – Lord Shiva
59. Faisal – Decisive
60. Gopal – Protector of cows
61. Himanshu – Moon
62. Inder – Lord Indra
63. Jagdish – Lord of the world
64. Karan – Helper
65. Lalit – Beautiful
66. Mohan – Charming
67. Naveen – New
68. Omkar – Another form of Lord Shiva
69. Pranay – Love

70. Raghav – Lord Rama
71. Sachin – Pure
72. Tejas – Brilliance
73. Ujjwal – Bright
74. Vivek – Wisdom
75. Yatin – Ascetic
76. Aniket – Lord of the world
77. Brijesh – Lord of Brij land
78. Chandan – Sandalwood
79. Devansh – Part of God
80. Eklavya – A student who learned by himself
81. Gaurav – Pride
82. Hitesh – Lord of goodness
83. Indrajit – Conqueror of Indra
84. Jayesh – Victor
85. Keshav – Another name for Lord Krishna
86. Manav – Human
87. Nishant – Dawn
88. Prabhat – Morning
89. Rishikesh – Lord Vishnu
90. Sanket – Signal
91. Tushar – Winter
92. Utsav – Celebration
93. Vaibhav – Richness
94. Yashpal – Protector of fame
95. Anshul – Sunbeam
96. Brij – Lord Krishna
97. Chintan – Contemplation
98. Devraj – King among gods
99. Ekansh – Whole
100. Gyan – Knowledge

Mexican baby boy names

1. Alejandro – Defender of mankind
2. Antonio – Priceless one
3. Carlos – Free man
4. Diego – Supplanter
5. Eduardo – Wealthy guardian
6. Fernando – Adventurous, brave traveler
7. Gabriel – God is my strength
8. Hector – Holding fast
9. Ignacio – Fiery
10. Javier – New house
11. Jose – God will increase
12. Juan – God is gracious
13. Luis – Famous warrior
14. Manuel – God is with us
15. Oscar – Divine spear
16. Pedro – Rock
17. Rafael – God has healed
18. Sergio – Servant
19. Victor – Conqueror
20. Miguel – Who is like God?
21. Ricardo – Powerful ruler
22. Rodrigo – Famous ruler
23. Enrique – Ruler of the household
24. Ramon – Wise protector
25. Francisco – Free man
26. Pablo – Small
27. Mario – Warlike
28. Julio – Youthful
29. Roberto – Bright fame
30. Andres – Manly, brave
31. Jesus – God is salvation
32. Felipe – Friend of horses
33. Ernesto – Serious, determined

34. Armando – Soldier
35. Ruben – Behold, a son
36. Gerardo – Spear rule
37. Guillermo – Will, desire, helmet, protection
38. Jorge – Farmer
39. Raul – Wolf counsel
40. Marcos – Warlike
41. Arturo – Bear
42. Alberto – Noble, bright
43. Angel – Messenger of God
44. Martin – Warlike
45. Gustavo – Staff of the gods
46. Alfonso – Noble and ready
47. Joaquin – Raised by God
48. Salvador – Savior
49. Rafael – God has healed
50. Emilio – Rival
51. Cesar – Long haired
52. Samuel – God has heard
53. Adan – Earth
54. Benito – Blessed
55. Bruno – Brown
56. Cristian – Follower of Christ
57. Daniel – God is my judge
58. David – Beloved
59. Esteban – Crown
60. Fabian – Bean grower
61. Felipe – Lover of horses
62. Gerardo – Spear brave
63. Hugo – Mind, intellect
64. Ismael – God will hear
65. Jaime – Supplanter
66. Leonardo – Brave lion
67. Mateo – Gift of God
68. Nicolas – Victory of the people
69. Orlando – Famous land

70. Patricio – Nobleman
71. Quirino – Spear
72. Ramiro – Judicious
73. Santiago – Saint James
74. Tomas – Twin
75. Uriel – God is my light
76. Valentino – Strength, health
77. Wilfredo – Desiring peace
78. Xavier – New house
79. Yago – Supplanter
80. Zacarias – God remembers
81. Abelardo – Noble, strong
82. Baltazar – God protect the king
83. Claudio – Lame
84. Dionisio – God of wine
85. Efrain – Fruitful
86. Faustino – Lucky
87. Gregorio – Watchful
88. Horacio – Timekeeper
89. Isidro – Gift of Isis
90. Jeronimo – Sacred name
91. Leandro – Lion man
92. Maximiliano – Greatest
93. Norberto – Bright north
94. Octavio – Eighth
95. Placido – Calm, quiet
96. Rogelio – Famous spear
97. Silvestre – Woods, forest
98. Teodoro – Gift of God
99. Ubaldo – Bold, brave
100. Virgilio – Flourishing

Brazilian baby boy names

1. Ademir – Noble protector
2. Adriano – Dark one
3. Alberto – Noble and bright
4. Alexandre – Defender of mankind
5. Alonzo – Noble and ready
6. Alvaro – Guardian
7. Andre – Warrior
8. Antonio – Priceless
9. Armando – Army man
10. Artur – Noble and courageous
11. Bernardo – Brave as a bear
12. Bruno – Brown
13. Caio – Rejoice
14. Carlos – Manly
15. Cesar – Hairy
16. Cristiano – Follower of Christ
17. Daniel – God is my judge
18. David – Beloved
19. Diego – Supplanter
20. Diogo – Doctrine
21. Eduardo – Wealthy guardian
22. Elias – The Lord is my God
23. Enrico – Ruler of the home
24. Estevao – Crown
25. Fabio – Bean grower
26. Felipe – Lover of horses
27. Fernando – Adventurous
28. Francisco – Free man
29. Gabriel – God is my strength
30. Guilherme – Helmet of will
31. Gustavo – Staff of the Goths
32. Henrique – Home ruler
33. Hugo – Mind, intellect

34. Igor – Warrior of peace
35. Isaac – Laughter
36. Joao – God is gracious
37. Jorge – Farmer
38. Jose – God will add
39. Juan – God is gracious
40. Julio – Youthful
41. Leonardo – Brave lion
42. Lucas – Light
43. Luis – Famous warrior
44. Manoel – God is with us
45. Marcelo – Little warrior
46. Marcos – Warlike
47. Mateus – Gift of God
48. Miguel – Who is like God?
49. Nuno – Ninth
50. Oscar – Divine spear
51. Paulo – Small
52. Pedro – Rock
53. Rafael – God has healed
54. Ramiro – Wise and famous
55. Ricardo – Powerful ruler
56. Roberto – Bright fame
57. Rodrigo – Famous ruler
58. Samuel – God has heard
59. Sergio – Servant
60. Thiago – Supplanter
61. Tomas – Twin
62. Vicente – Conquering
63. Vitor – Conqueror
64. Wagner – Wagon-maker
65. Xavier – New house
66. Yago – Supplanter
67. Zane – God is gracious
68. Abel – Breath
69. Acacio – The Lord holds

70. Bento – Blessed
71. Ciro – Sun
72. Dario – Wealthy
73. Eneas – Praise
74. Fausto – Lucky
75. Geraldo – Ruler with a spear
76. Horacio – Timekeeper
77. Inacio – Fiery
78. Jaco – Supplanter
79. Lino – A cry of grief
80. Nilo – From the Nile
81. Otavio – Eighth
82. Paco – Free
83. Quirino – Spear
84. Raul – Wise wolf
85. Silvio – Wood
86. Tito – Giant
87. Ugo – Heart, mind, and spirit
88. Vasco – Crow
89. Xico – Free man
90. Yuri – Farmer
91. Zacarias – The Lord has remembered
92. Iago – Supplanter
93. Olavo – Ancestor's descendent
94. Heitor – To hold or possess
95. Jair – He shines
96. Kaua – Rejoice
97. Levi – Joined in harmony
98. Noel – Born on Christmas
99. Uriel – God is my light
100. Valentim – Healthy, strong

Russian baby boy names

1. Aleksandr - Defender of mankind
2. Anatoliy - Sunrise
3. Andrey - Manly, brave
4. Anton - Priceless one
5. Arkadiy - From Arcadia
6. Arseniy - Virile, potent
7. Artur - Bear
8. Boris - Fighter, warrior
9. Danil - God is my judge
10. Dmitriy - Earth-lover
11. Eduard - Wealthy guardian
12. Evgeniy - Well born
13. Fyodor - God's gift
14. Gavriil - God is my strength
15. Georgiy - Farmer
16. Grigoriy - Watchful, alert
17. Igor - Warrior of peace
18. Ilya - The Lord is my God
19. Ivan - God is gracious
20. Kirill - Lordly, master's
21. Konstantin - Steadfast
22. Kuzma - Universe
23. Leonid - Lion's son
24. Lev - Lion
25. Maksim - Greatest
26. Mikhail - Who is like God?
27. Nikita - Unconquered
28. Nikolay - People's victory
29. Oleg - Holy, blessed
30. Pavel - Small, humble
31. Pyotr - Rock, stone
32. Roman - From Rome
33. Sergey - Servant

34. Stanislav - Fame, glory
35. Stepan - Crown, garland
36. Timofey - Honouring God
37. Valentin - Healthy, strong
38. Vasily - Royal, kingly
39. Vladislav - Rule with glory
40. Vladimir - Famous ruler
41. Yaroslav - Spring glory
42. Yegor - Farmer
43. Yuriy - Farmer
44. Zakhar - God has remembered
45. Zinoviy - Life of Zeus
46. Rodion - Song of the hero
47. Mark - Warlike
48. Alexey - Defender
49. Semyon - God has heard
50. Vsevolod - Ruler of all
51. Matvey - Gift of God
52. Vadim - Ruler
53. Yuliy - Youthful
54. Khariton - Grace, kindness
55. Rostislav - Usurp glory
56. Innokentiy - Innocent
57. Gleb - Godly life
58. Prokhor - Leader of the dance
59. Miroslav - Peace and glory
60. Taras - Of Tarentum
61. Platon - Broad-shouldered
62. Savva - Old man
63. Marat - Dedicated to Mars
64. Filipp - Lover of horses
65. German - Brother
66. Tikhon - Lucky, fortunate
67. Radomir - Happy peace
68. Luka - Light
69. Yaromir - Spring peace

70. Venedikt - Blessed
71. Naum - Comforter
72. Klim - Merciful
73. Leon - Lion
74. Yulian - Youthful
75. Yakov - Supplanter
76. Roland - Famous throughout the land
77. Samuil - God has heard
78. Rodion - Hero's song
79. Ruslan - Lion man
80. Viktor - Conqueror
81. Fedor - Gift of God
82. Erik - Eternal ruler
83. Vasil - King
84. Emelyan - Rival
85. Denis - God of wine
86. David - Beloved
87. Artem - Safe, sound
88. Albert - Noble, bright
89. Adam - Man
90. Yefim - Well-spoken
91. Nestor - Homecoming
92. Modest - Moderate
93. Makar - Blessed
94. Lazar - God has helped
95. Kliment - Merciful, gentle
96. Iosif - He will add
97. Ignat - Fiery
98. Gerasim - Old age
99. Efrem - Fruitful
100. Afanasiy - Immortal

Dutch baby boy names

1. Aart - Noble, brave
2. Abel - Breath, vapour
3. Adrian - Dark one
4. Albert - Noble, bright
5. Alexander - Defender of the people
6. Andre - Brave, manly
7. Anton - Priceless one
8. Arjen - Bright, shining
9. Barend - Bear brave
10. Bastiaan - Revered
11. Benjamin - Son of the right hand
12. Bert - Bright, shining
13. Bram - Father of a multitude
14. Casper - Treasurer
15. Christiaan - Follower of Christ
16. Cornelis - Horn
17. Daan - God is my judge
18. Diederik - Ruler of the people
19. Dirk - Ruler of the people
20. Edvard - Wealthy guardian
21. Evert - Strong as a boar
22. Floris - Flower
23. Frans - Free man
24. Gerard - Brave with a spear
25. Gijs - Bright pledge
26. Hans - God is gracious
27. Hendrik - Ruler of the home
28. Hugo - Mind, intellect
29. Isaac - He will laugh
30. Jacob - Supplanter
31. Jan - God is gracious
32. Jasper - Treasurer
33. Jeroen - Holy name

34. Joost - Just, fair
35. Kees - Horn
36. Koen - Bold advisor
37. Lars - Crowned with laurel
38. Leendert - Brave as a lion
39. Lucas - Light
40. Maarten - Warlike
41. Mark - Warlike
42. Matthijs - Gift of God
43. Michiel - Who is like God?
44. Nick - Victory of the people
45. Oscar - Divine spear
46. Paul - Small, humble
47. Peter - Rock
48. Pieter - Rock
49. Quinten - Fifth
50. Rens - Laurel
51. Roel - Famous land
52. Rutger - Famous spear
53. Sander - Defender of mankind
54. Sebastiaan - Revered
55. Simon - He has heard
56. Stefan - Crown
57. Teun - Priceless
58. Theo - God's gift
59. Thomas - Twin
60. Tim - Honouring God
61. Tobias - God is good
62. Victor - Conqueror
63. Vincent - Conquering
64. Willem - Will, desire
65. Wouter - Ruler of the army
66. Xander - Defender of mankind
67. Yannick - God is gracious
68. Yves - Yew, bow army
69. Zacharias - God has remembered

70. Zeger - Victory bearer
71. Felix - Happy, fortunate
72. Gerardus - Brave with a spear
73. Johannes - God is gracious
74. Jurgen - Farmer
75. Laurens - Crowned with laurel
76. Leonardus - Brave as a lion
77. Maxim - The greatest
78. Olivier - Olive tree
79. Reinier - Deciding warrior
80. Thijs - Gift of God
81. Arnoud - Eagle power
82. Berend - Bear brave
83. Emiel - Rival
84. Frederik - Peaceful ruler
85. Gregor - Watchful, alert
86. Hendrick - Home ruler
87. Ivar - Bow warrior
88. Karel - Free man
89. Leopold - Bold people
90. Marius - Male, virile
91. Norbert - Bright north
92. Otto - Wealth, fortune
93. Pim - Will, desire
94. Quintin - Fifth
95. Roderick - Famous power
96. Sjoerd - Guard
97. Ties - Gift of God
98. Uri - My light
99. Valentijn - Strong, healthy
100. Wessel - Army vessel

Swedish baby boy names

1. Adam – Man, Earth
2. Adrian – From Hadria
3. Albin – White, Bright
4. Alexander – Defender of mankind
5. Alfred – Elf counselor
6. Anders – Strong, Manly
7. Anton – Priceless
8. Arne – Eagle
9. Axel – Father of peace
10. Benjamin – Son of the right hand
11. Bjorn – Bear
12. Carl – Free man
13. Christian – Follower of Christ
14. Daniel – God is my judge
15. David – Beloved
16. Edvin – Rich friend
17. Elias – The Lord is my God
18. Emil – Rival
19. Erik – Eternal ruler
20. Filip – Lover of horses
21. Fredrik – Peaceful ruler
22. Gabriel – God is my strength
23. Gustav – Staff of the Gods
24. Hannes – God is gracious
25. Henrik – Home ruler
26. Hugo – Mind, Intellect
27. Isak – He will laugh
28. Jakob – Supplanter
29. Johan – God is gracious
30. Jonas – Dove
31. Karl – Free man
32. Kasper – Treasurer
33. Kevin – Handsome

34. Kim – Chief, Ruler
35. Lars – Laurel
36. Leif – Heir, Descendant
37. Linus – Flaxen
38. Lucas – Light
39. Ludvig – Famous warrior
40. Magnus – Great
41. Marcus – Warlike
42. Martin – Warlike
43. Mathias – Gift of God
44. Max – Greatest
45. Mikael – Who is like God?
46. Nils – Champion
47. Olof – Ancestor's heir
48. Oscar – Friend of deer
49. Otto – Wealth, Fortune
50. Patrik – Nobleman
51. Paul – Small
52. Peter – Rock
53. Pontus – Sea
54. Rasmus – Beloved
55. Robert – Bright fame
56. Roger – Famous spear
57. Rolf – Famous wolf
58. Samuel – God has heard
59. Sebastian – Venerable
60. Simon – He has heard
61. Stefan – Crown
62. Stig – Wanderer
63. Sven – Boy, Lad
64. Tobias – God is good
65. Tomas – Twin
66. Ulf – Wolf
67. Viktor – Conqueror
68. Vilhelm – Will, Desire, Helmet
69. Vincent – Conquering

70. William – Resolute protector
71. Yngve – God of the Ingwaz
72. Zacharias – God has remembered
73. Aage – Ancestor
74. Aksel – Father of peace
75. Knut – Knot
76. Leif – Heir, Descendant
77. Njord – Strong, Vigorous
78. Ragnar – Army, Warrior
79. Sigurd – Guardian of victory
80. Tor – Thunder
81. Ulrik – Prosperity, Power
82. Valdemar – Famous ruler
83. Ingmar – Famous son
84. Jesper – Treasurer
85. Joakim – Raised by God
86. Kjell – Kettle, Helmet
87. Lennart – Lion, Brave
88. Mårten – Warlike
89. Niklas – Victory of the people
90. Oskar – Friend of deer
91. Per – Rock
92. Rune – Secret
93. Staffan – Crown
94. Tord – Thor's thunder
95. Viggo – War
96. Åke – Ancestor
97. Örjan – Farmer
98. Göran – Farmer
99. Håkan – High son
100. Ingvar – Warrior of Ing

Norwegian baby boy names

1. Aksel - Father of Peace
2. Bjorn - Bear
3. Christian - Follower of Christ
4. Dag - Day
5. Erik - Ever Ruler
6. Finn - From Finland
7. Gustav - Staff of the Gods
8. Hakon - High Son
9. Ingvar - Warrior of Ing
10. Johan - God is Gracious
11. Karl - Free Man
12. Lars - Crowned with Laurels
13. Magnus - Great
14. Nils - People's Victory
15. Olav - Ancestor's Descendant
16. Per - Rock
17. Roald - Famous Ruler
18. Sven - Boy
19. Tore - Thunder God
20. Ulf - Wolf
21. Vidar - Wide Warrior
22. Yngve - Son of Ing
23. Alf - Elf Counsel
24. Bjarne - Bear
25. Canute - Knot
26. Dagfinn - Day Finder
27. Einar - One Warrior
28. Frode - Wise
29. Geir - Spear
30. Halvard - Rock Guardian
31. Isak - He Laughs
32. Jens - God is Gracious
33. Knut - Knot

34. Leif -   Heir
35. Mathias -   Gift of God
36. Odd -   Point of a Sword
37. Peder -   Rock
38. Ragnar -   Army Rule
39. Sigurd -   Guardian of Victory
40. Tor -   Thunder
41. Ulrik -   Prosperity and Power
42. Vilhelm -   Resolute Protector
43. Ystein -   Island Stone
44. Anders -   Manly
45. Brage -   Poet
46. Casper -   Treasurer
47. Daniel -   God is my Judge
48. Edvard -   Wealthy Guardian
49. Gabriel -   God is my Strength
50. Harald -   Army Ruler
51. Ivar -   Bow Warrior
52. Jakob -   Supplanter
53. Kjell -   Kettle
54. Ludvig -   Famous Warrior
55. Mikkel -   Who is like God
56. Oscar -   Friend of Deer
57. Peter -   Rock
58. Rasmus -   Beloved
59. Sigmund -   Victorious Protector
60. Tobias -   God is Good
61. Valdemar -   Famous Ruler
62. William -   Resolute Protector
63. Adam -   Man
64. Benjamin -   Son of the Right Hand
65. Christopher -   Bearer of Christ
66. David -   Beloved
67. Elias -   Yahweh is God
68. Filip -   Friend of Horses
69. Henrik -   Home Ruler

70. Jonas - Dove
71. Kim - Ruler
72. Markus - Warlike
73. Noah - Rest
74. Oskar - Friend of Deer
75. Paul - Small
76. Ruben - Behold, a Son
77. Sebastian - Venerable
78. Thomas - Twin
79. Victor - Conqueror
80. Adrian - From Hadria
81. Alexander - Defender of the People
82. Caspar - Treasurer
83. Emil - Rival
84. Felix - Lucky
85. Hugo - Mind, Intellect
86. Isaac - He Laughs
87. Julian - Youthful
88. Liam - Resolute Protector
89. Maximilian - Greatest
90. Oliver - Olive Tree
91. Rafael - God has Healed
92. Simon - He has Heard
93. Tristan - Tumult
94. Vincent - Conquering
95. Zacharias - Yahweh Remembers
96. Anton - Priceless One
97. Bernard - Brave as a Bear
98. Dominic - Belonging to the Lord
99. Frederick - Peaceful Ruler
100. Gregory - Watchful, Alert

Danish baby boy names

1. Aage - Honored, respected
2. Aksel - Father of peace
3. Anders - Manly, brave
4. Anker - Manly, brave
5. Arne - Eagle
6. Asger - Spear of God
7. Axel - Father of peace
8. Bendt - Blessed
9. Bjarke - Bear
10. Bjorn - Bear
11. Carsten - Christian
12. Christian - Follower of Christ
13. Claus - Victory of the people
14. Dag - Day
15. Einar - One warrior
16. Emil - Rival
17. Erik - Eternal ruler
18. Esben - Bear
19. Finn - Fair
20. Frederik - Peaceful ruler
21. Gorm - He who worships god
22. Gregers - Watchful, alert
23. Gunnar - Warrior
24. Gustav - Staff of the gods
25. Hakon - High son
26. Hans - God is gracious
27. Harald - Army ruler
28. Henrik - Home ruler
29. Herluf - Wolf
30. Ib - Yew
31. Ingvar - Warrior of Ing
32. Jakob - Supplanter
33. Jens - God is gracious

34. Jeppe - Supplanter
35. Joergen - Farmer
36. Johan - God is gracious
37. Jonas - Dove
38. Jorgen - Farmer
39. Jorn - Farmer
40. Kai - Rejoice
41. Karsten - Christian
42. Keld - Spring, fountain
43. Kjeld - Helmet, protection
44. Knud - Knot
45. Lars - Crowned with laurel
46. Leif - Heir, descendant
47. Lennart - Lion strength
48. Magnus - Great
49. Mogens - Power
50. Morten - From the god Mars
51. Nels - Champion
52. Niels - Champion
53. Nils - Champion
54. Olaf - Ancestor's descendant
55. Ole - Ancestor's descendant
56. Orjan - Farmer
57. Osvald - God's power
58. Otto - Wealth
59. Peder - Rock
60. Per - Rock
61. Preben - First battle
62. Rasmus - Beloved
63. Roar - Famous spear
64. Rune - Secret
65. Soren - Severe
66. Steen - Stone
67. Sten - Stone
68. Svend - Boy, lad
69. Sven - Boy, lad

70. Tage - Day
71. Thor - Thunder
72. Thorkild - Thunder, helmet
73. Torben - Thunder, bear
74. Troels - Thor's arrow
75. Ulf - Wolf
76. Ulrik - Wolf power
77. Valdemar - Famous power
78. Viggo - War
79. Vilhelm - Will, desire and helmet, protection
80. Vagn - Wagon
81. Aaren - Enlightened
82. Abel - Breath
83. Abell - Breath
84. Adalbert - Noble, bright
85. Adelbert - Noble, bright
86. Adolf - Noble wolf
87. Adolph - Noble wolf
88. Aksell - Father of peace
89. Albrekt - Noble, bright
90. Alek - Defender of mankind
91. Algot - Noble Geat
92. Alrik - All-powerful ruler
93. Ambrosius - Immortal
94. Anbjorn - Eagle bear
95. Anker - Manly
96. Ansgar - Spear of God
97. Anton - Priceless
98. Arild - Eagle power
99. Arvid - Eagle tree
100. Asmund - Divine protection

Finnish baby boy names

1. Aapo - Father of many nations
2. Aarne - Eagle
3. Aarno - Eagle power
4. Aatos - Thought
5. Ahti - Rich or generous
6. Aimo - Generous amount
7. Aki - Bright, shining
8. Aleksanteri - Defender of mankind
9. Altti - Noble, bright
10. Anssi - God is gracious
11. Antero - Manly, brave
12. Antti - Priceless
13. Armas - Dear, beloved
14. Arto - Bear
15. Asko - Divine reward
16. Atte - Father-like
17. Eeli - The Lord is my God
18. Eemeli - Rival
19. Eero - Eternal ruler
20. Eetu - Wealthy guardian
21. Eino - Lone warrior
22. Elias - The Lord is my God
23. Eljas - The Lord is my God
24. Ensio - First one
25. Erkki - Ever ruler
26. Esko - God-bear
27. Hannu - God is gracious
28. Harri - Home ruler
29. Heikki - Home ruler
30. Heimo - Tribe, home
31. Heino - House owner
32. Hemmo - Home
33. Henri - Home ruler

34. Iiro - Watchful, vigilant
35. Iisakki - He will laugh
36. Ilari - Cheerful, happy
37. Ilmari - Air
38. Ilpo - Air
39. Immo - World mighty
40. Isto - Stone
41. Jaakko - Supplanter
42. Jalmari - Helmeted warrior
43. Jani - God is gracious
44. Jari - Helmeted warrior
45. Jarkko - Earth worker
46. Jarmo - Helmeted warrior
47. Jere - God will uplift
48. Jesse - Gift
49. Jiri - Earth worker
50. Joakim - Raised by God
51. Joonas - Dove
52. Jooseppi - He will add
53. Jorma - Farmer
54. Juhani - God is gracious
55. Juho - God is gracious
56. Jukka - God is gracious
57. Jussi - God is gracious
58. Kaapo - God's messenger
59. Kalle - Free man
60. Kari - Pure
61. Karri - Pure
62. Keijo - Gentle, noble
63. Kerkko - Church-goer
64. Kimmo - Brave warrior
65. Kuisma - Beauty, order
66. Kustaa - Staff of the gods
67. Lari - Laurel-crowned
68. Lauri - Laurel-crowned
69. Leevi - Joined, attached

70. Lenni - Brave as a lion
71. Markku - Warlike
72. Martti - Warlike
73. Matias - God's gift
74. Matti - God's gift
75. Mika - Who is like God?
76. Mikko - Who is like God?
77. Nuutti - Wealthy, fortunate
78. Oiva - Excellent
79. Olavi - Ancestor's descendant
80. Onni - Happiness, luck
81. Oskari - God's spear
82. Otto - Wealth, fortune
83. Paavo - Small, humble
84. Panu - Fire
85. Pekka - Stone, rock
86. Pentti - Fifth
87. Pertti - Bright, famous
88. Petri - Stone, rock
89. Pietari - Stone, rock
90. Pirkka - Noble, distinguished
91. Raimo - Protecting hands
92. Risto - Christ-bearer
93. Sakari - God remembers
94. Sami - Listener
95. Seppo - Smith
96. Tapio - God of the forest
97. Teppo - God's honor
98. Timo - Honoring God
99. Toivo - Hope
100. Valtteri - Ruler of the army

Greek baby boy names

1. Achilles – Hero from the Iliad
2. Adonis – Beautiful
3. Aeneas – To praise
4. Aesop – Uncertain, possibly from Ethiopia
5. Agathos – Good
6. Ajax – Eagle
7. Alekos – Defender of mankind
8. Alexandros – Defender of mankind
9. Andreas – Manly
10. Angelos – Messenger
11. Apollo – Destroyer
12. Aristos – Best
13. Arsenios – Virile
14. Athanasios – Immortal
15. Bion – Life
16. Chariton – Grace, kindness
17. Chrysanthos – Golden flower
18. Cleon – Glorious
19. Cosmas – Order, decency
20. Damianos – To tame
21. Darius – Possessor of good
22. Demetrios – Follower of Demeter
23. Dionysios – Follower of Dionysus
24. Doros – Gift
25. Efthymios – Happy
26. Eleftherios – Free
27. Elias – My God is Yahweh
28. Eros – Love
29. Eudoros – Generous gift
30. Eustachios – Fruitful
31. Evander – Good man
32. Fotios – Light
33. Georgios – Farmer

34. Gerasimos – Old age
35. Gregorios – Watchful, alert
36. Hector – To hold, to possess
37. Helios – Sun
38. Herakles – Glory of Hera
39. Hermes – Messenger
40. Hesiod – To send song
41. Hieronymos – Sacred name
42. Hippolytos – Freer of horses
43. Homer – Hostage
44. Hyakinthos – Hyacinth flower
45. Iason – Healer
46. Ikaros – Follower
47. Ioannis – God is gracious
48. Isidoros – Gift of Isis
49. Kallistos – Most beautiful
50. Konstantinos – Constant, steadfast
51. Kostas – Constant, steadfast
52. Kyros – Lord
53. Leon – Lion
54. Leandros – Lion of a man
55. Linos – Flax
56. Lukas – From Lucania
57. Lysandros – Liberator
58. Makarios – Blessed
59. Melanthios – Black flower
60. Menelaus – Withstanding the people
61. Michail – Who is like God?
62. Nestor – Homecoming
63. Nikolaos – Victory of the people
64. Odysseus – Wrathful
65. Orestes – Mountain man
66. Orion – Boundary, limit
67. Panagiotis – All-holy
68. Panteleimon – All-compassionate
69. Paris – Wager

70. Perseus – To destroy
71. Petros – Stone
72. Philippos – Friend of horses
73. Platon – Broad, flat
74. Polys – Much
75. Pyrrhos – Flame-coloured, red
76. Sevastianos – Venerable
77. Sokrates – Power
78. Spyros – Spirit
79. Stephanos – Crown
80. Stavros – Cross
81. Stylianos – Pillar
82. Tassos – Harvester
83. Telemachos – Far from battle
84. Theodoros – Gift of god
85. Theophilos – Friend of god
86. Theron – Hunter
87. Theseus – To set
88. Timotheos – Honouring god
89. Titos – White clay, honourable
90. Vasileios – King
91. Xanthos – Yellow, blonde
92. Xenophon – Strange voice
93. Xerxes – Ruler over heroes
94. Zephyros – West wind
95. Zeno – Of Zeus
96. Zeus – Sky, shine
97. Zoticus – Life-giving
98. Agapetos – Beloved
99. Anastasios – Resurrection
100. Sotirios – Saviour

Turkish baby boy names

1. Ahmet - Highly praised or one who constantly thanks God
2. Ali - Noble, sublime
3. Mustafa - The chosen one
4. Osman - Tender youth
5. Mehmet - Praised one
6. Hasan - Good, beautiful
7. Hüseyin - Small beauty
8. Selim - Safe, undamaged
9. İbrahim - Father of many
10. Yusuf - God will add
11. Murat - Wish, desire
12. Ömer - Life, long living
13. Emir - Command, prince
14. Cem - Ruler, king
15. Deniz - Sea
16. Can - Life, soul
17. Barış - Peace
18. Aydın - Enlightened, intellectual
19. Erol - Brave man
20. Fatih - Conqueror
21. Gökhan - Sky, ruler
22. Harun - Exalted, high mountain
23. İsmail - God will hear
24. Kerem - Noble, generous
25. Levent - Handsome, good-looking
26. Mert - Brave, gallant
27. Nihat - Clean, pure
28. Onur - Honor, pride
29. Polat - Steel
30. Raşit - Rightly guided
31. Serhat - Border
32. Taha - Pure, innocent

33. Ufuk - Horizon
34. Vedat - Love, affection
35. Yakup - Supplanter
36. Zeki - Intelligent, clever
37. Adil - Just, fair
38. Bülent - High, lofty
39. Cihan - Universe, cosmos
40. Devrim - Revolution
41. Engin - Broad, widespread
42. Ferit - Unique, incomparable
43. Gürkan - Strong, firm
44. Hakan - Emperor, ruler
45. İlhan - Prince, noble
46. Kemal - Perfection, integrity
47. Lütfullah - Grace of God
48. Mesut - Happy, lucky
49. Nuri - My fire, my light
50. Orhan - Leader, ruler
51. Recep - Welcoming, hospitable
52. Sami - Elevated, sublime
53. Taner - Dawn man
54. Umut - Hope
55. Veli - Guardian, protector
56. Yasin - Prophet's name
57. Zülküf - One of the prophets
58. Arda - He who comes from the bottom
59. Bilal - Water, freshness
60. Cemal - Beauty
61. Doğan - Falcon
62. Erdem - Virtue, morality
63. Fikret - Thought, idea
64. Gökçe - Sky blue
65. Halil - Close friend
66. İzzet - Honor, respect
67. Kadir - Powerful, capable
68. Mahir - Skilled, proficient

69. Necati - Beneficial, useful
70. Okan - Heart, mind
71. Rıza - Consent, satisfaction
72. Selçuk - A historical Turkish tribe
73. Tuncay - Bronze moon
74. Uğur - Good luck, fortune
75. Volkan - Volcano
76. Yılmaz - Indomitable, undefeatable
77. Zafer - Victory, triumph
78. Atilla - Father-like
79. Burak - Bright, shining
80. Cenk - Battle, war
81. Durmuş - He has stopped
82. Ender - Very rare
83. Fuat - Heart, mind
84. Gürbüz - Strong, healthy young man
85. Haldun - Forever, eternal
86. İdris - To instruct, to study
87. Kaan - Prince, lord
88. Metin - Strong, firm
89. Nurettin - Light of the religion
90. Oktay - Taurus moon
91. Reha - Free, liberated
92. Sinan - Spearhead
93. Tayfun - Typhoon
94. Ufuk - Horizon
95. Vedat - Affection, love
96. Yavuz - Grim, stern
97. Ziya - Light, splendor
98. Asım - Protector, guardian
99. Berke - Hard, tough
100. Cüneyt - Little soldier

Egyptian baby boy names

1. Aadam - It man or earth
2. Abasi - It signifies stern or serious
3. Abdul - It servant of God
4. Abydos - A name of a city in ancient Egypt
5. Adio - It righteous
6. Akhenaten - It effective spirit of Aten
7. Akil - It signifies intelligent or thoughtful
8. Amasis - It born of the moon
9. Amenhotep - It peace of Amon
10. Ammon - It the hidden one
11. Anubis - It royal child
12. Asim - It signifies protector or guardian
13. Ata - It twin
14. Aten - It sun disk
15. Ayman - It signifies blessed or lucky
16. Azibo - It earth
17. Badru - It born during the full moon
18. Bakari - It signifies one who will succeed
19. Bakt - It to be satisfied or full
20. Cairo - Named after the capital city of Egypt
21. Dakarai - It signifies happiness
22. Darius - It to possess
23. Djoser - It the most sacred one
24. Fenuku - It signifies born late
25. Gamal - It beauty or elegance
26. Gahiji - It signifies a hunter
27. Haji - It one born during the pilgrimage
28. Hasani - It signifies handsome
29. Horus - It god of light
30. Imhotep - It the one who comes in peace
31. Isis - It throne
32. Jabari - It signifies brave
33. Jahi - It dignified

34. Jamal - It signifies beauty
35. Jamil - It signifies handsome
36. Jengo - It building
37. Kafele - It signifies worth dying for
38. Kamuzu - It medical
39. Kek - It god of darkness
40. Kepher - It to transform
41. Khafra - It signifies appearing like Ra
42. Khufu - It signifies protected by the god Khnum
43. Maahes - It lion
44. Makalani - It signifies a palm tree
45. Malik - It signifies king
46. Mekal - It signifies fierce devourer
47. Menes - It signifies established
48. Menna - It signifies a good man
49. Merenre - It signifies lover of Re
50. Minkah - It signifies justice
51. Mobarak - It signifies blessed
52. Mosi - It signifies firstborn
53. Naeem - It signifies comfort
54. Nahar - It signifies day
55. Naji - It signifies safe
56. Nefertum - It signifies young Atum
57. Nekhbet - It signifies she of Nekheb
58. Nkosi - It signifies ruler
59. Nomti - It signifies strong
60. Obasi - It signifies in honor of the supreme god
61. Osiris - It signifies with strong eyesight
62. Panya - It signifies mouse
63. Pili - It signifies second-born
64. Ptah - It signifies creator
65. Qeb - It signifies the earth
66. Ra - It signifies sun
67. Ramesses - It signifies born of Ra
68. Rashidi - It signifies wise
69. Razi - It signifies secret

70. Rehema - It signifies merciful
71. Sabola - It signifies prophet
72. Sefu - It signifies sword
73. Sekani - It signifies laughter
74. Seti - It signifies of Seth
75. Shabaka - It signifies king
76. Sobek - It signifies crocodile
77. Tahir - It signifies pure
78. Tawfiq - It signifies success
79. Thutmose - It signifies born of Thoth
80. Tutankhamun - It signifies living image of Amun
81. Umi - It signifies life
82. Unas - It signifies king
83. Usi - It signifies smoke
84. Wamukota - It signifies god of rain
85. Xola - It signifies stay in peace
86. Yafeu - It signifies bold
87. Zahur - It signifies flower
88. Zalika - It signifies well-born
89. Zesiro - It signifies first-born twin
90. Zuberi - It signifies strong
91. Zuri - It signifies beautiful
92. Zwi - It signifies gazelle
93. Keket - It signifies goddess of darkness
94. Khonsu - It signifies traveler
95. Ma'at - It signifies truth
96. Nefertiti - It signifies a beautiful woman has come
97. Nekhen - It signifies hawk city
98. Osaze - It signifies loved by God
99. Qaletaqa - It signifies guardian of the people
100. Ram - It signifies high, supreme

South African baby boy names

1. Aiden - little fire
2. Akhona - present
3. Bandile - they have multiplied
4. Caleb - whole-hearted
5. Dingaan - praiseworthy
6. Ethan - strong
7. Fana - adoration
8. Gcobani - be joyful
9. Hlumelo - root
10. Iminathi - God is with us
11. Jabulani - be happy
12. Khaya - home
13. Lethabo - happiness
14. Mthunzi - shade
15. Nkosi - king
16. Onke - enough
17. Phakama - rise
18. Qhawe - hero
19. Rethabile - we are happy
20. Sipho - gift
21. Thabo - joy
22. Unathi - God is with us
23. Vuyo - happiness
24. Wanda - desirable
25. Xolani - peace
26. Yonela - enough
27. Zola - quiet
28. Andile - increase
29. Bongani - be thankful
30. Cyprian - from Cyprus
31. Dumisani - praise
32. Emihle - beautiful
33. Fikile - arrived

34. Gugulethu - our treasure
35. Hlanganani - unite
36. Inathi - God is with us
37. Jomo - burning spear
38. Khulani - grow
39. Lungelo - right
40. Mzwandile - the family has increased
41. Nkosana - little king
42. Oarabile - he has done for us
43. Phumzile - rest
44. Qinisela - persevere
45. Rorisang - praise
46. Sanele - we are satisfied
47. Thulani - be quiet
48. Uzile - satisfied
49. Vusumuzi - bring back life
50. Wandile - increased
51. Xhanti - patience
52. Yanga - admire
53. Zwide - wide
54. Ayabonga - thank you
55. Bhekizizwe - look after the nation
56. Cebisa - advise
57. Dabulamanzi - divider of the waters
58. Emile - industrious
59. Fundile - it is complete
60. Gcinumuzi - preserve the household
61. Hlomla - respect
62. Iniko - born during troubled times
63. Jengo - one with red skin
64. Kwanda - increase
65. Luvuyo - joy
66. Mandla - power
67. Ntando - will
68. Olwethu - our own
69. Phakade - forever

70. Qaphela - be careful
71. Rethabile - we are happy
72. Sandile - we have extended
73. Thando - love
74. Ukhona - he is present
75. Vumile - agree
76. Wakhile - he has built
77. Xola - stay in peace
78. Yibanathi - be with us
79. Zweli - country
80. Ayize - let it happen
81. Bonginkosi - thank the Lord
82. Cebo - gift
83. Daluxolo - peace maker
84. Enzokuhle - do good
85. Fuzo - reflection
86. Gcina - keep
87. Hlubi - good
88. Inam - God's favor
89. Jengo - one with red skin
90. Kwanele - it is enough
91. Lwandle - ocean
92. Mandlenkosi - power of God
93. Ntando - will
94. Olwethu - our own
95. Phumelelo - success
96. Qaqamba - intelligent
97. Radebe - we have become more numerous
98. Sakhile - we have built
99. Thamsanqa - luck
100. Uzile - satisfied

Nigerian baby boy names

1. Ade - Royal or Crown
2. Chijioke - God's gift
3. Obi - Heart
4. Chike - God's power
5. Uche - Thought or Will
6. Ifeanyi - Nothing is impossible with God
7. Chidi - God is there
8. Emeka - Great deeds
9. Chukwuemeka - God has done great
10. Okechukwu - God's gift
11. Olumide - My God has come
12. Oluwaseun - Thank God
13. Abiodun - Born during a festival
14. Babatunde - Father has returned
15. Olufemi - God loves me
16. Olusegun - God is victorious
17. Segun - Conqueror
18. Tunde - The returned one
19. Akin - Hero or Brave one
20. Femi - Love me
21. Gbenga - Lift up
22. Kola - Wealth
23. Yemi - Respect me
24. Dele - Come home
25. Adeola - Crown of wealth
26. Bolaji - Awake in wealth
27. Ola - Wealth
28. Jide - Arrive
29. Olu - God
30. Kayode - He who brings joy
31. Dotun - Became sweet
32. Ayo - Joy
33. Bayo - Joy has found us

34. Dayo - Joy arrives
35. Wale - Come home
36. Dapo - Join together
37. Olakunle - Wealth fills the house
38. Olanrewaju - My wealth is the future
39. Olugbenga - God lifts up
40. Opeyemi - I give thanks
41. Taiwo - Taste the world
42. Kehinde - The one who came after
43. Idris - Studious person
44. Kabir - Great
45. Lateef - Gentle
46. Raheem - Merciful
47. Tariq - Morning star
48. Yusuf - God will add
49. Akeem - Wise
50. Azeez - Respected
51. Basir - Wise
52. Fola - Honor
53. Jameel - Handsome
54. Kareem - Generous
55. Malik - King
56. Nasir - Helper
57. Rafiq - Friend
58. Sani - Brilliant
59. Zain - Beautiful
60. Abubakar - Noble
61. Mukhtar - Chosen
62. Mustapha - The chosen one
63. Nuhu - Rest or Comfort
64. Umar - Long-lived
65. Yakubu - God will protect
66. Zayd - To prosper
67. Habib - Beloved
68. Ibrahim - Father of many
69. Ismail - God will hear

70. Jibril - God is my strength
71. Salim - Safe
72. Tijani - Crown or Diadem
73. Uthman - Baby bustard
74. Yusuf - God increases
75. Jamal - Beauty
76. Rashid - Rightly guided
77. Samir - Companion in evening talk
78. Tahir - Pure
79. Wasi - Broad-minded
80. Yasin - Prophet's name
81. Zahir - Shining or Radiant
82. Amin - Trustworthy
83. Farouk - One who distinguishes truth from falsehood
84. Hakim - Wise
85. Idris - Interpreter
86. Jabir - Comforter
87. Khalid - Eternal
88. Lutfi - Kind
89. Munir - Shining
90. Nabil - Noble
91. Qasim - Divider
92. Rais - Captain
93. Sule - Asked for
94. Tawfiq - Success
95. Uzair - Helper
96. Wahid - Unique
97. Yasir - Wealthy
98. Zafir - Victorious
99. Aqil - Intelligent
100. Badr - Full moon

Kenyan baby boy names

1. Adongo - Firstborn of twins
2. Akoko - Time of birth
3. Baraka - Blessing
4. Chacha - Strong
5. Chege - Scholar
6. Daudi - Beloved
7. Ebo - Born on Tuesday
8. Fadhili - Kindness or generosity
9. Gakuo - Elder
10. Habari - News or message
11. Imara - Strong or resolute
12. Jengo - Building
13. Kamau - Quiet warrior
14. Kito - Precious child
15. Lekan - My wealth is growing
16. Madaraka - Independence or freedom
17. Njau - Bull
18. Ochieng - Born when the sun shines
19. Pili - Second born
20. Raha - Happiness or joy
21. Sefu - Sword
22. Tendaji - Makes things happen
23. Ujana - Youth
24. Vumbi - Dust
25. Wachira - Son of a trader
26. Yaro - Son
27. Zuberi - Strong
28. Amani - Peace
29. Balozi - Ambassador
30. Chike - Power of God
31. Dera - Home
32. Enzi - Powerful
33. Faraji - Comfort

34. Gamba - Warrior
35. Haki - Justice
36. Imani - Faith
37. Jengo - Building
38. Kibwe - Blessed
39. Lengo - Goal or aim
40. Makena - Happy one
41. Nia - Purpose
42. Odongo - Second of twins
43. Penda - Love
44. Rafiki - Friend
45. Safari - Journey
46. Taji - Crown
47. Umoja - Unity
48. Wanyonyi - Born during the weeding season
49. Zawadi - Gift
50. Abasi - Serious
51. Bahari - Sea
52. Chane - Dependable
53. Dunia - Earth
54. Eshe - Life
55. Faruq - Discerning truth from falsehood
56. Gwamaka - Well-known
57. Hasani - Handsome
58. Iniko - Born during troubled times
59. Jengo - Building
60. Kofi - Born on Friday
61. Lutalo - Warrior
62. Moseka - Fire
63. Njoro - Farmer
64. Onyango - Born at dawn
65. Panya - Mouse
66. Rama - Pleasing
67. Simba - Lion
68. Tumaini - Hope
69. Usia - Born during famine

70. Wema - Goodness
71. Zuri - Beautiful
72. Azibo - Earth
73. Bwana - Lord or master
74. Chuma - Wealth
75. Daktari - Doctor
76. Enzi - Powerful
77. Fumo - Ninth-born child
78. Gamba - Warrior
79. Hekima - Wisdom
80. Isaya - God is my salvation
81. Jengo - Building
82. Kito - Jewel
83. Liko - Born during the farming season
84. Mchumba - Sweetheart
85. Nuru - Light
86. Ojwang - Born during the harvesting season
87. Pili - Second
88. Rais - President
89. Sisi - Born on Sunday
90. Tano - Fifth-born child
91. Usama - Lion
92. Wendo - Love
93. Zalika - Well-born
94. Ayo - Joy
95. Binti - Daughter
96. Chiku - Chatterer
97. Doto - The younger of twins
98. Esiankiki - Young maiden
99. Furaha - Joy
100. Gitonga - Rich in possessions

Ghanaian baby boy names

1. Kwabena - Born on Tuesday
2. Kofi - Born on Friday
3. Kwame - Born on Saturday
4. Kwaku - Born on Wednesday
5. Yaw - Born on Thursday
6. Kojo - Born on Monday
7. Ekow - Born on Thursday
8. Kwasi - Born on Sunday
9. Nana - King or monarch
10. Akwasi - Born on Sunday
11. Kwadwo - Born on Monday
12. Akwetey - Second born son
13. Paa - Good
14. Ebo - Born on Tuesday
15. Kwabla - Born on Tuesday
16. Kwamena - Born on Saturday
17. Ato - Born on Wednesday
18. Akoto - Second born after twins
19. Amo - Born on Saturday
20. Kweku - Born on Wednesday
21. Kwao - Born on Monday
22. Kobena - Born on Tuesday
23. Kwadwo - Born on Monday
24. Kobby - Born on Tuesday
25. Fiifi - Born on Friday
26. Yaw - Born on Thursday
27. Ekua - Born on Wednesday
28. Nii - King or superior
29. Kakra - Second born child
30. Obi - Heart
31. Adom - Blessing or grace
32. Agyenim - God's wisdom
33. Kyei - Dignity

34. Osei - Noble or honorable
35. Ohene - King or ruler
36. Bonsu - Whale, symbolizing greatness
37. Gyamfi - Adventurous
38. Antwi - First born of a set of twins
39. Boakye - Adventurer
40. Frimpong - Strong man
41. Amankwah - Greatness
42. Akenten - Bravery or courage
43. Asante - Grateful
44. Appiah - Prince or nobleman
45. Acheampong - Destined for greatness
46. Owusu - Strong-willed and determined
47. Opoku - Humble and virtuous
48. Prempeh - Adventurous
49. Afrifa - Born during war
50. Agyei - Messenger of God
51. Danso - Reliable
52. Ababio - Child that keeps coming back
53. Nyamekye - God's gift
54. Agyapong - Noble
55. Adjei - Eagle, symbolizing strength
56. Adu - First child of a second husband
57. Ankomah - Journey of life
58. Ameyaw - Praise God
59. Badu - Tenth-born child
60. Boamah - Strong-willed
61. Bempah - Fifth-born child
62. Botwe - Third-born child
63. Donkor - Humble
64. Domfeh - Reliable
65. Gyasi - Wonderful
66. Kwarteng - Ninth-born child
67. Kusi - Happy
68. Oteng - Tree, symbolizing strength
69. Ofori - A helper

70. Poku - Humble
71. Sarpong - Supreme
72. Twum - Twin
73. Yamoah - God's gift
74. Yeboah - God's gift
75. Zuta - Helper
76. Amoah - Strength of God
77. Ahenkan - First child after twins
78. Boaten - King of the golden stool
79. Kwansah - Second son after twins
80. Nyantakyi - Seventh-born child
81. Ofori-Atta - Helper and brave
82. Okyere - Teacher or counselor
83. Owusu-Ansah - God's servant
84. Prah - Savior
85. Quansah - God's gift
86. Sakyi - Mighty or powerful
87. Takyi - Brave
88. Wiredu - Knowledgeable
89. Yeboah - God's gift
90. Adu-Boahen - First child of a second husband, brave
91. Agyapong - Noble
92. Amponsah - Destined for greatness
93. Boadu - Adventurous
94. Effah - Seventh-born child
95. Gyamfi - Adventurous
96. Kyei - Dignity
97. Nyarko - Seventh-born child
98. Opoku - Humble and virtuous
99. Sarfo - Charitable
100. Tweneboah - God's gift

Ethiopian baby boy names

1. Abebe -   he has blossomed
2. Abinet -   he has appeared
3. Abiy -   my father
4. Abreham -   father of many
5. Adane -   their son
6. Adisu -   new beginning
7. Afework -   speaks pleasant things
8. Alem -   world
9. Alemayehu -   I have seen the world
10. Amare -   he is handsome
11. Andargachew -   you are the crown
12. Asfaw -   the coming of the sun
13. Asrat -   blessing
14. Ayele -   he has become strong
15. Bahir -   sea
16. Bekele -   to grow
17. Berhanu -   his light
18. Binyam -   son of the south
19. Chernet -   become my strength
20. Dagnachew -   my pillar
21. Daniel -   God is my judge
22. Dawit -   beloved
23. Dejen -   foundation
24. Demisse -   peace
25. Desta -   joy
26. Ermias -   God has uplifted
27. Eskinder -   the first man
28. Fasil -   castle
29. Fekadu -   my longing
30. Fikre -   my love
31. Fitsum -   my silence
32. Gabre -   servant of God
33. Gashaw -   my love

34. Gebre - servant
35. Geremew - he is my guardian
36. Getachew - his master
37. Getahun - my lord
38. Girma - he is respected
39. Haile - power
40. Hailu - his power
41. Henock - dedicated
42. Iyasu - Jesus
43. Jember - his sunset
44. Kaleb - faithful
45. Kebede - my servant
46. Kedir - capable
47. Kidane - my covenant
48. Kifle - my property
49. Lij - child
50. Mamo - my relative
51. Mekonnen - the angel
52. Melaku - his angel
53. Mengistu - government
54. Mesfin - his boundary
55. Meskel - cross
56. Mikael - who is like God
57. Mulu - complete
58. Natnael - God has given
59. Nebiyu - prophet
60. Negus - king
61. Nigus - emperor
62. Petros - rock
63. Redda - he has helped
64. Saba - morning
65. Selam - peace
66. Semere - he is my joy
67. Senay - good news
68. Seyoum - he is my comfort
69. Tadesse - he has been reborn

70. Tamirat -   he is health
71. Tariku -   he is history
72. Tasfaye -   my hope
73. Teferi -   he is my respect
74. Tekle -   plant
75. Teklu -   he is my planting
76. Tewodros -   gift of God
77. Tilahun -   he is my time
78. Walelign -   he is above
79. Wondimu -   his brother
80. Workneh -   you are gold
81. Yared -   he is descent
82. Yohannes -   God is gracious
83. Yonas -   dove
84. Zelalem -   eternal
85. Zerihun -   he is a seed
86. Zewedu -   his crown
87. Amanuel -   God is with us
88. Assefa -   he has cleared
89. Biruk -   he is blessed
90. Chala -   best
91. Dereje -   he has become smart
92. Eyoel -   God is my strength
93. Frew -   fruit
94. Girma -   he is respected
95. Habtamu -   he is rich
96. Ibsa -   he has opened
97. Jemal -   beauty
98. Kassahun -   he has divided
99. Leul -   prince
100. Mekuria -   his kingdom

Moroccan baby boy names

1. Aahil – Prince
2. Aariz – Respectable man
3. Abdul – Servant of God
4. Adil – Just, Honest
5. Ahmed – Highly praised
6. Akram – Generous
7. Ali – Exalted, Noble
8. Amine – Faithful, Trustworthy
9. Anas – Affection, Love
10. Ayman – Lucky, Right-handed
11. Bilal – Water, Freshness
12. Badr – Full Moon
13. Basim – Smiling
14. Chafik – Sympathetic
15. Daoud – Beloved
16. Driss – Star
17. Ehab – Gift
18. Fadil – Generous, Honorable
19. Farid – Unique, Singular
20. Ghali – Valuable
21. Hakim – Wise, Judicious
22. Hamza – Strong, Firm
23. Harun – Mountain
24. Ibrahim – Father of a multitude
25. Idris – A Prophet's name
26. Ismail – God will hear
27. Jamal – Beauty
28. Jawad – Generous
29. Kader – Powerful
30. Karim – Generous, Noble
31. Khalid – Eternal
32. Lamine – Trustworthy
33. Malik – King

34. Marwan – Solid
35. Mohammed – Praised
36. Mustafa – Chosen
37. Nabil – Noble
38. Nizar – Little
39. Omar – Long-lived
40. Othman – Companion of Prophet Muhammad
41. Rachid – Rightly guided
42. Rafik – Friend
43. Said – Happy
44. Salah – Righteousness
45. Samir – Entertaining companion
46. Tariq – Morning star
47. Walid – Newborn
48. Yahya – God is gracious
49. Yasin – Prophet's name
50. Youssef – God will add
51. Zaid – Increase, Growth
52. Zaki – Pure
53. Zakaria – God remembers
54. Ziyad – Abundance
55. Abbas – Lion
56. Abdu – Servant of God
57. Adnan – Settler
58. Aqil – Intelligent
59. Asad – Lion
60. Aziz – Powerful, Beloved
61. Baha – Beautiful, Brilliant
62. Bashar – Bringer of glad tidings
63. Dahir – Evident, Clear
64. Eisa – The Arabic name for Jesus
65. Faisal – Judge, Decisive
66. Galal – Greatness
67. Hadi – Guide to righteousness
68. Hamid – Praiseworthy
69. Hassan – Handsome

70. Ilyas – The Lord is my God
71. Imad – Support, Pillar
72. Jafar – Little Stream
73. Kamal – Perfection
74. Khalil – Friend
75. Latif – Gentle, Kind
76. Majid – Noble, Glorious
77. Nasim – Breeze
78. Qasim – Divider
79. Rauf – Merciful
80. Sabir – Patient
81. Talal – Nice, Admirable
82. Umar – Life
83. Waleed – Newborn
84. Yaqub – Supplanter
85. Yusuf – God will add
86. Zahir – Bright, Shining
87. Zuhair – Bright, Shining
88. Fakhri – Honorary
89. Ihab – Leather
90. Jalal – Majesty
91. Kabir – Great
92. Luqman – Wise
93. Munir – Luminous, Enlightening
94. Nuh – Rest, Peace
95. Qadir – Capable
96. Raed – Leader
97. Sami – Elevated, Sublime
98. Tawfiq – Success, Reconciliation
99. Ubaid – Faithful
100. Yasir – Wealthy

Algerian baby boy names

1. Abdel - servant of God
2. Adel - righteous
3. Ahmed - highly praised
4. Ali - exalted
5. Amine - faithful
6. Anis - friendly
7. Ayoub - Job, the prophet
8. Bakir - early
9. Bilal - water
10. Chafik - sympathetic
11. Djamal - beauty
12. Elias - God is my Lord
13. Fadil - generous
14. Farid - unique
15. Ghani - rich
16. Hakim - wise
17. Idris - interpreter
18. Jamal - beauty
19. Karim - generous
20. Latif - gentle
21. Malik - king
22. Nabil - noble
23. Omar - flourishing
24. Qadir - capable
25. Rafik - friend
26. Saad - happiness
27. Tariq - morning star
28. Umar - long life
29. Wahid - unique
30. Yasin - prophet's name
31. Zaki - pure
32. Hamza - lion
33. Ilyas - the Lord is my God

34. Jibril - God is my strength
35. Khalil - friend
36. Marwan - solid
37. Nawfal - generous
38. Qasim - one who distributes
39. Rami - archer
40. Sabri - patient
41. Taha - A title of the Prophet Muhammad
42. Wael - seeker
43. Youssef - God will add
44. Zakaria - God has remembered
45. Harun - exalted
46. Imad - pillar
47. Jalil - great
48. Khaled - eternal
49. Mounir - luminous
50. Nour - light
51. Rahim - merciful
52. Sami - elevated
53. Tawfiq - success
54. Walid - newborn
55. Yacine - rich
56. Zaid - growth
57. Hicham - generosity
58. Ismail - God will hear
59. Jihad - struggle
60. Kamal - perfection
61. Mustafa - chosen
62. Nizar - small
63. Rached - guided
64. Sofiane - pure
65. Tayeb - kind
66. Wassim - handsome
67. Yassir - easy
68. Zine - beauty
69. Hani - happy

70. Issa - God is salvation
71. Kais - firm
72. Lounis - companion
73. Moussa - saved from the water
74. Nadjib - intelligent
75. Rachid - rightly guided
76. Salah - righteousness
77. Tarik - morning star
78. Yacoub - supplanter
79. Yassine - prosperous
80. Zahir - shining
81. Habib - beloved
82. Jalel - majesty
83. Kamil - perfect
84. Lotfi - kind
85. Mokhtar - chosen
86. Nafis - precious
87. Rafiq - friend
88. Salim - safe
89. Toufik - good luck
90. Yahya - God is gracious
91. Yazed - God will increase
92. Zouhir - flower
93. Hakem - ruler
94. Jalal - greatness
95. Kamel - complete
96. Madjid - glorious
97. Nouri - light
98. Ramzi - symbolic
99. Samir - companion in evening talk
100. Youssef - God will increase

Tunisian baby boy names

1. Aadam - Man of Earth
2. Aamir - Prosperous or full of life
3. Aban - Old Arabic name
4. Abbas - Stern or lion
5. Abdul - Servant of God
6. Adel - Just or fair
7. Adnan - Settler
8. Ahmed - Highly praised
9. Akram - Most generous
10. Ammar - Long-lived
11. Anis - Companion or friend
12. Arif - Knowledgeable
13. Asad - Lion
14. Ashraf - Most noble
15. Ayman - Lucky
16. Aziz - Powerful
17. Badr - Full moon
18. Bashar - Bringer of good news
19. Bassam - Smiling
20. Bilal - Water
21. Burhan - Proof
22. Daoud - Beloved
23. Dhafer - Victorious
24. Ehab - Gift
25. Fahd - Lynx
26. Faisal - Resolute
27. Farid - Unique
28. Fathi - Conqueror
29. Fouad - Heart
30. Ghassan - Youth
31. Habib - Beloved
32. Hadi - Guide
33. Hafid - Descendant

34. Hakim - Wise
35. Hamid - Praiseworthy
36. Hamza - Steadfast
37. Haroun - High mountain
38. Hassan - Handsome
39. Hichem - Generous
40. Hisham - Generous
41. Idris - Studious
42. Imad - Support
43. Ismail - God will hear
44. Iyad - Support
45. Jamal - Beauty
46. Jawad - Generous
47. Jihad - Struggle
48. Kais - Firm
49. Kamal - Perfection
50. Karim - Generous
51. Khalid - Eternal
52. Khayri - Charitable
53. Lamine - Trustworthy
54. Lotfi - Gentle
55. Mahdi - Guided one
56. Mahmoud - Praised
57. Majdi - Glorious
58. Mansour - Victorious
59. Marouane - Solid
60. Moez - Honorable
61. Mohamed - Praised
62. Moussa - Saved from the water
63. Mounir - Shining
64. Nabil - Noble
65. Nader - Rare
66. Najib - Noble
67. Nasr - Victory
68. Nizar - Little
69. Nour - Light

70. Omar - Life
71. Othman - Companion of Prophet Muhammad
72. Rabah - Winner
73. Rachid - Rightly guided
74. Raed - Pioneer
75. Rafik - Friend
76. Rami - Archer
77. Ramzi - Symbolic
78. Rashad - Good sense
79. Rayan - Watered
80. Riad - Garden
81. Sabri - Patient
82. Saif - Sword
83. Salim - Safe
84. Sami - High, elevated
85. Samir - Entertaining companion
86. Sofiane - Pure
87. Taha - A chapter of the Quran
88. Tariq - Morning star
89. Walid - Newborn
90. Wassim - Handsome
91. Yahya - God is gracious
92. Yasin - A chapter of the Quran
93. Youssef - God will increase
94. Zahir - Bright
95. Zaki - Pure
96. Ziad - Abundance
97. Zine - Beauty
98. Ziyad - Growth
99. Zubair - Strong, firm
100. Zuhair - Bright

Libyan baby boy names

1. Aban - Old Arabic name
2. Abdul - Servant of God
3. Adel - Fair, Just
4. Ahmad - Highly praised
5. Akram - Most generous
6. Ali - Noble, High
7. Ammar - Long-lived
8. Anas - Affection, love
9. Aqil - Intelligent
10. Arif - Knowing, aware
11. Asad - Lion
12. Ashraf - Most noble
13. Ayman - Lucky
14. Aziz - Powerful, respected
15. Badr - Full moon
16. Basim - Smiling
17. Bilal - Water, freshness
18. Daud - Beloved
19. Faisal - Decisive
20. Farid - Unique
21. Fathi - Conqueror
22. Ghazi - Conqueror
23. Hadi - Guide
24. Hamid - Praised
25. Hamza - Lion
26. Harun - Exalted, noble
27. Hasan - Handsome
28. Hatim - Judge
29. Hisham - Generous
30. Ibrahim - Father of a multitude
31. Idris - Studious
32. Imad - Pillar, support
33. Ismail - God will hear

34. Jamal - Beauty
35. Jibril - God is my strength
36. Karim - Generous
37. Khalid - Eternal
38. Khayri - Charitable
39. Latif - Gentle, kind
40. Luqman - Wise
41. Mahdi - Guided one
42. Mahmud - Praiseworthy
43. Majid - Glorious
44. Malik - King
45. Mansur - Victorious
46. Marwan - Solid
47. Masud - Fortunate
48. Moez - Honorable
49. Muhsin - Beneficent
50. Mustafa - Chosen one
51. Nabil - Noble
52. Nader - Rare
53. Nasir - Helper
54. Omar - Flourishing, long-lived
55. Qasim - Divider
56. Rafiq - Friend
57. Rahim - Merciful
58. Rashid - Rightly guided
59. Rayan - Luxuriant
60. Rida - Contentment
61. Sabir - Patient
62. Salah - Righteousness
63. Samir - Entertainer
64. Sayid - Master
65. Shakir - Thankful
66. Sulaiman - Peaceful
67. Tariq - Morning star
68. Umar - Flourishing, long-lived
69. Usman - Baby bustard

70. Wael - Seeker of refuge
71. Walid - Newborn
72. Yasin - The opening letters of Surah 36 in the Qur'an
73. Youssef - God will increase
74. Zaid - Increase, growth
75. Zaki - Pure
76. Ziyad - Growth, abundance
77. Aazim - Determined
78. Badri - One who took part in the battle of Badr
79. Fakhr - Pride, glory
80. Ghassan - Youth, prime of life
81. Hafiz - Guardian, protector
82. Hashim - Destroyer of evil
83. Ihsan - Beneficence
84. Jahan - World
85. Karam - Generosity
86. Lutfi - Kind, friendly
87. Mubarak - Blessed
88. Nasr - Victory
89. Qadir - Powerful
90. Rafi - High, exalted
91. Sajid - One who prostrates
92. Taha - A name of the Prophet Muhammad
93. Ubaid - Small slave
94. Wajih - Noble
95. Yasir - Wealthy
96. Zuhair - Bright, shining
97. Bahir - Dazzling, brilliant
98. Da'ud - Beloved
99. Faiz - Victorious
100. Jabir - Comforter, bringer of consolation

Saudi Arabian baby boy names

1. Abdullah - servant of God
2. Abdulrahman - servant of the merciful
3. Ahmed - praised or praiseworthy
4. Ali - exalted or noble
5. Amir - prince or ruler
6. Ayman - right hand or blessed
7. Bashar - bringer of good news
8. Bilal - water
9. Faisal - decisive or resolute
10. Fahad - panther or leopard
11. Faris - knight or horseman
12. Hamza - strong or steadfast
13. Hassan - handsome or good
14. Hussein - handsome or beautiful
15. Ibrahim - father of many
16. Idris - interpreter
17. Jamal - beauty
18. Khaled - eternal or immortal
19. Malik - king or owner
20. Mohammed - praiseworthy
21. Mustafa - chosen one
22. Nasser - helper or supporter
23. Omar - flourishing or long-lived
24. Qasim - one who distributes
25. Rashid - rightly guided
26. Saad - good luck
27. Salman - safe or secure
28. Tariq - morning star
29. Waleed - newborn
30. Yasser - wealthy
31. Zaid - to increase
32. Zayn - beauty or grace
33. Adel - righteous

34. Badr - full moon
35. Essam - safeguard
36. Ghassan - youth or strength
37. Haris - guardian or protector
38. Ihab - gift
39. Jafar - stream
40. Karim - generous or noble
41. Latif - gentle or kind
42. Mubarak - blessed
43. Nabil - noble or generous
44. Qadir - capable or powerful
45. Rafiq - friend or companion
46. Sabir - patient
47. Tahir - pure or clean
48. Ubaid - servant of God
49. Yahya - alive or living
50. Zakir - one who remembers
51. Asad - lion
52. Basim - smiling
53. Daoud - beloved
54. Emir - commander or prince
55. Fadi - savior
56. Ghazi - warrior
57. Hadi - guide
58. Imad - pillar or support
59. Jalal - majesty
60. Kamal - perfection
61. Luqman - wise
62. Muhannad - sword
63. Nawaf - high, lofty
64. Qusay - distant
65. Raed - pioneer
66. Sami - elevated or sublime
67. Talal - admirable
68. Usama - lion
69. Yaqub - supplanter

70. Zuhair - little flower
71. Atif - compassionate
72. Bahir - dazzling
73. Dhiya - light
74. Fakhr - pride
75. Ghalib - victor
76. Habib - beloved
77. Ihsan - charity or benevolence
78. Jalil - great or revered
79. Karam - generosity
80. Lutfi - kind
81. Muhsin - beneficent
82. Nadir - rare
83. Qahtan - ancient
84. Ra'uf - merciful
85. Sadiq - truthful
86. Tamim - complete
87. Umar - flourishing or thriving
88. Yasin - rich
89. Ziyad - growth
90. Azzam - determined
91. Bilal - moisture
92. Dabir - teacher
93. Fawaz - successful
94. Ghayth - rain
95. Hashim - destroyer of evil
96. Ilyas - the Lord is my God
97. Jibril - God is my strength
98. Khalil - friend
99. Majid - glorious
100. Nuh - comforter or rest

Iranian baby boy names

1. Aban - Old Arabic name
2. Abtin - A character in Shahnameh
3. Adel - Righteous
4. Adib - Cultured, well-mannered
5. Afshin - A character in Shahnameh
6. Aftab - The sun
7. Ahmad - Highly praised
8. Akbar - Greater, bigger
9. Ali - Exalted, noble
10. Alireza - Name of Prophet Muhammad's grandson
11. Amjad - More glorious
12. Anahita - Immaculate
13. Anoush - Immortal
14. Arash - A hero in Persian folklore
15. Ardeshir - A character in Shahnameh
16. Arman - Hope, wish
17. Armin - A character in Shahnameh
18. Arsalan - Lion
19. Artin - Righteous
20. Ashkan - A character in Shahnameh
21. Aslan - Lion
22. Ata - Gift
23. Azad - Free
24. Babak - Little father
25. Bahman - Good mind
26. Bahram - A character in Shahnameh
27. Bijan - A character in Shahnameh
28. Borzou - A character in Shahnameh
29. Cyrus - Sun
30. Dara - Wealthy
31. Davood - Beloved
32. Ehsan - Charity
33. Emad - Pillar

34. Esfandiar - A character in Shahnameh
35. Faraz - Above
36. Farbod - Right, orthodox
37. Farid - Unique
38. Farshad - Happy
39. Farzad - Splendid birth
40. Fereydoun - A character in Shahnameh
41. Garshasp - A character in Shahnameh
42. Giv - A character in Shahnameh
43. Hafez - Guardian
44. Hamid - Praiseworthy
45. Hashem - Name of Prophet Muhammad's grandfather
46. Hassan - Handsome
47. Hossein - Handsome
48. Iraj - A character in Shahnameh
49. Jahan - World
50. Jamshid - A character in Shahnameh
51. Javad - Generous
52. Kambiz - Fortunate
53. Kamran - Successful
54. Karim - Generous
55. Kaveh - A character in Shahnameh
56. Kayvan - World, universe
57. Kian - Kings
58. Kourosh - Like the sun
59. Mani - A painter who later claimed to be a prophet
60. Manuchehr - A character in Shahnameh
61. Maziar - Devoted to the Mazdayasna religion
62. Mehran - Kindness
63. Milad - Birth
64. Mobin - Clear, evident
65. Mohammad - Praised one
66. Morteza - Chosen one
67. Nader - Rare
68. Navid - Good news

69. Omid - Hope
70. Parviz - Victorious
71. Payam - Message
72. Pedram - Lucky
73. Pejman - Grieved
74. Pirouz - Victorious
75. Pouya - Seeker
76. Ramin - A character in Shahnameh
77. Reza - Will, consent
78. Rostam - A character in Shahnameh
79. Saeed - Happy
80. Saman - Home
81. Shahab - Shooting star
82. Shahin - Falcon
83. Shahram - A character in Shahnameh
84. Shapour - A character in Shahnameh
85. Siavash - A character in Shahnameh
86. Soheil - Name of a star
87. Sohrab - A character in Shahnameh
88. Taha - A Surah in Quran
89. Taher - Pure
90. Vahid - Unique
91. Varun - God of water in Hindu mythology
92. Yaghoub - Name of a prophet
93. Yahya - Name of a prophet
94. Yasin - A Surah in Quran
95. Yousef - God will multiply
96. Zal - A character in Shahnameh
97. Zartosht - Golden star
98. Zia - Light
99. Ziya - Light
100. Zohrab - A character in Shahnameh

Iraqi baby boy names

1. Abdullah - Servant of God
2. Ahmed - The praised one
3. Akram - Most Generous
4. Ali - Exalted, Noble
5. Amir - Prince, Commander
6. Anwar - Light
7. Aqeel - Wise, Intelligent
8. Arif - Knowledgeable, Learned
9. Asif - Gather, Harvest
10. Ayman - Lucky, Righteous
11. Aziz - Powerful, Beloved
12. Badr - Full moon
13. Bahir - Dazzling, Brilliant
14. Basim - Smiling
15. Bilal - Water, Moisture
16. Daoud - Beloved, Friend
17. Dinar - Gold coin
18. Emir - Commander, Prince
19. Fadi - Redeemer, Savior
20. Faisal - Judge, Decisive
21. Farid - Unique, Singular
22. Farouk - Truthful
23. Fawzi - Successful, Victorious
24. Ghazi - Conqueror, Warrior
25. Hadi - Guide to righteousness
26. Hakim - Wise, Ruler
27. Hamid - Praiseworthy
28. Haris - Guardian, Protector
29. Hasan - Handsome, Good
30. Hussein - Handsome, Beautiful
31. Ibrahim - Father of many
32. Idris - Studious, Knowledgeable
33. Imad - Pillar, Support

34. Ismail - God will hear
35. Jamal - Beauty
36. Jawad - Generous, Open-handed
37. Kadir - Capable, Competent
38. Karim - Generous, Noble
39. Khalid - Eternal, Immortal
40. Khayrat - Good deeds, Charitable acts
41. Latif - Kind, Gentle
42. Mahdi - Guided to the right path
43. Mahmud - Praiseworthy
44. Majid - Noble, Glorious
45. Malik - King, Owner
46. Mansour - Victorious
47. Marwan - Solid, Quartz
48. Moeen - Helper, Supporter
49. Mufid - Useful, Beneficial
50. Mustafa - Chosen One
51. Nabil - Noble, Generous
52. Nadir - Rare, Precious
53. Naji - Safe, Survivor
54. Nasir - Helper, Protector
55. Omar - Long-lived, Flourishing
56. Qasim - Divider, Distributor
57. Rafiq - Kind, Gentle
58. Rahim - Merciful, Compassionate
59. Rashid - Rightly guided, Mature
60. Rauf - Compassionate, Kind
61. Rida - Contentment, Satisfaction
62. Saad - Happiness, Good fortune
63. Sabir - Patient, Persevering
64. Salim - Safe, Sound
65. Sami - High, Exalted
66. Sharif - Noble, Honorable
67. Tahir - Pure, Clean
68. Talib - Seeker, Student
69. Tariq - Morning star, Knocker

70. Umar - Life, Long living
71. Usman - Baby bustard
72. Waleed - Newborn
73. Yahya - God is gracious
74. Yasin - Prophet's name
75. Youssef - God will increase
76. Zafir - Victorious
77. Zahir - Bright, Shining
78. Zaki - Pure, Chaste
79. Ziad - Abundance, Growth
80. Amin - Trustworthy, Honest
81. Samir - Entertaining companion
82. Ihab - Gift
83. Rami - Archer
84. Firas - Perspicacity
85. Iyad - Reinforcement
86. Adnan - Settler
87. Hayder - Lion
88. Muhsin - Beneficent
89. Badir - Full moon
90. Suhail - Easy, Uncomplicated
91. Luqman - Wise
92. Jafar - Rivulet, Stream
93. Hisham - Generous
94. Qadir - Powerful, Capable
95. Sajjad - Prostrating in prayer
96. Tawfiq - Success, Reconciliation
97. Zain - Beauty, Grace
98. Nizar - Little
99. Yaqub - Supplanter
100. Zakariya - God has remembered

Israeli baby boy names

1. Aaron – High mountain
2. Abdiel – Servant of God
3. Abraham – Father of many
4. Adam – Man, Earth
5. Adir – Great, mighty
6. Aharon – Light bringer
7. Aiden – Little fire
8. Akiva – Protect, shelter
9. Amos – Carried by God
10. Ari – Lion
11. Ariel – Lion of God
12. Asher – Happy
13. Avi – My father
14. Aviv – Spring
15. Barak – Lightning
16. Ben – Son
17. Benjamin – Son of the right hand
18. Caleb – Devotion to God
19. Chaim – Life
20. Daniel – God is my judge
21. David – Beloved
22. Doron – Gift
23. Efraim – Fruitful
24. Eli – High, ascended
25. Elijah – My God is Yahweh
26. Eliezer – My God is help
27. Erez – Cedar tree
28. Ethan – Firm, enduring
29. Ezra – Help
30. Gabriel – God is my strength
31. Gideon – Feller, hewer
32. Gil – Joy, happiness
33. Haim – Life

34. Isaac – He will laugh
35. Isaiah – Salvation of the Lord
36. Ishai – Gift
37. Israel – Contend with God
38. Jacob – Supplanter
39. Jair – He shines
40. Jaron – Singing
41. Jedidiah – Beloved of the Lord
42. Jesse – Gift
43. Jonathan – God has given
44. Joseph – He will add
45. Joshua – God is salvation
46. Judah – Praised
47. Kaleb – Whole hearted
48. Levi – Joined, attached
49. Liam – Resolute protector
50. Liron – My joy
51. Malachi – My messenger
52. Matan – Gift
53. Micah – Who is like God
54. Michael – Who is like God
55. Moshe – Drawn out of the water
56. Nathan – He gave
57. Nathaniel – God has given
58. Noah – Rest, comfort
59. Oded – Encourager
60. Omer – Sheaf of wheat
61. Ori – My light
62. Orin – Light
63. Raphael – God has healed
64. Reuben – Behold, a son
65. Ron – Song, joy
66. Samson – Sun
67. Samuel – God has heard
68. Saul – Asked for, prayed for
69. Shai – Gift

70. Shalom – Peace
71. Shimon – He has heard
72. Solomon – Peace
73. Tamar – Date palm tree
74. Uri – My light
75. Uriel – God is my light
76. Uzi – My strength
77. Yaakov – Supplanter
78. Yael – Mountain goat
79. Yair – He will enlighten
80. Yaniv – He will prosper
81. Yaron – Singing
82. Yehuda – Praised
83. Yeshua – Salvation
84. Yigal – He will redeem
85. Yitzhak – He will laugh
86. Yoav – The Lord is father
87. Yochanan – God is gracious
88. Yonatan – God has given
89. Yosef – He will add
90. Yotam – God is perfect
91. Zev – Wolf
92. Zion – Highest point
93. Zohar – Light, brilliance
94. Zvi – Deer, gazelle
95. Eitan – Strong and steadfast
96. Eyal – Strength
97. Nissim – Miracles
98. Itai – Friendly
99. Tal – Dew
100. Noam – Pleasantness, charm

Palestinian baby boy names

1. Ahmad - Praiseworthy, commendable
2. Akram - Generous
3. Amir - Prince, commander
4. Anas - Affection, love
5. Ayman - Lucky, right-handed
6. Bashar - Bringer of good news
7. Bassam - Smiling
8. Bilal - Refreshing
9. Fadi - Redeemer, savior
10. Farid - Unique, precious
11. Ghassan - Youth, prime of life
12. Hadi - Guide, leader
13. Hamza - Lion
14. Idris - Interpreter
15. Imran - Prosperity, happiness
16. Ismail - God will hear
17. Jamal - Beauty, grace
18. Khaled - Eternal
19. Laith - Lion
20. Majid - Noble, glorious
21. Nabil - Noble, wise
22. Omar - Life, long-lived
23. Qasim - Divider, distributor
24. Rashid - Rightly guided
25. Samir - Entertaining companion
26. Tariq - Morning star
27. Usama - Lion
28. Wael - Seeker of refuge
29. Yahya - God is gracious
30. Ziad - Abundance, growth
31. Adnan - Settler
32. Baha - Splendor, glory
33. Daoud - Beloved

34. Emad - Support, pillar
35. Faisal - Decisive
36. Ghalib - Conqueror
37. Habib - Beloved
38. Ihab - Gift
39. Jalal - Majesty, glory
40. Kamal - Perfection, integrity
41. Latif - Gentle, kind
42. Munir - Luminous, shining
43. Nasir - Helper, protector
44. Osman - Servant of God
45. Qadir - Capable, powerful
46. Raed - Leader
47. Salim - Safe, sound
48. Tamim - Complete, perfect
49. Umar - Flourishing, thriving
50. Yasin - Rich, prosperous
51. Zain - Beauty, grace
52. Abdul - Servant of God
53. Bilal - Moisture
54. Da'ud - Beloved
55. Elias - The Lord is my God
56. Fawaz - Successful
57. Ghazi - Warrior
58. Hakim - Wise
59. Ilyas - The Lord is my God
60. Jamal - Beauty
61. Karim - Generous
62. Lutfi - Kind, gentle
63. Mustafa - Chosen one
64. Nizar - Little
65. Othman - Baby bustard
66. Qusay - Distant
67. Rafiq - Gentle, friend
68. Saif - Sword
69. Taha - Pure

70. Uthman - Companion of the Prophet
71. Yasir - Wealthy
72. Zahir - Bright, shining
73. Abdullah - Servant of God
74. Bashar - Bringer of glad tidings
75. Dawood - Beloved
76. Fahad - Lynx
77. Ghaffar - Forgiving
78. Hashim - Destroyer of evil
79. Ibrahim - Father of a multitude
80. Jafar - Stream
81. Khalid - Immortal
82. Malik - King
83. Naeem - Comfort, ease
84. Omar - Long life
85. Qais - Firm
86. Rashad - Good sense, maturity
87. Salah - Righteousness
88. Tariq - Morning star
89. Usaid - Small lion
90. Yaqub - Supplanter
91. Zaki - Pure
92. Abdur - Servant of God
93. Bilal - Conqueror
94. Daud - Beloved
95. Faisal - Resolute
96. Ghayth - Rain
97. Hassan - Handsome
98. Iqbal - Prosperity
99. Jalal - Glory
100. Kareem - Noble, generous

Jordanian baby boy names

1. Abdullah – Servant of God
2. Ahmed – Highly praised
3. Ali – Exalted, Noble
4. Amir – Prince, Commander
5. Ayman – Lucky, Right-handed
6. Bashar – Bringer of Good News
7. Bilal – Water, Moisture
8. Daoud – Beloved
9. Faisal – Decisive, Judge
10. Faris – Horseman, Knight
11. Ghassan – Youth, Prime of life
12. Habib – Beloved
13. Hadi – Guide to righteousness
14. Idris – Studious, Learned
15. Imran – Prosperity, Happiness
16. Jamal – Beauty
17. Kamil – Perfect, Complete
18. Karim – Generous, Noble
19. Latif – Gentle, Kind
20. Majid – Noble, Glorious
21. Nabil – Noble, Generous
22. Omar – Long-lived
23. Qasim – Divider, Distributor
24. Raed – Leader
25. Samir – Entertainer
26. Tariq – Morning star
27. Yasin – Prophet's name
28. Zaid – Increase, Growth
29. Adnan – Settler
30. Basim – Smiling
31. Fahd – Leopard
32. Hamza – Steadfast, Lion
33. Ihab – Gift

34. Jafar – Stream
35. Kamal – Perfection
36. Luay – Shield
37. Murad – Desired
38. Nizar – Bright, Glowing
39. Osman – Servant of God
40. Qadir – Capable, Powerful
41. Rami – Archer
42. Sufyan – Fast walker
43. Talal – Admirable
44. Waleed – Newborn
45. Yasir – Wealthy
46. Ziyad – Increase, Growth
47. Amin – Trustworthy
48. Bishr – Joy
49. Fadi – Redeemer
50. Hani – Happy, Delighted
51. Ibrahim – Father of a multitude
52. Jalal – Greatness
53. Khalid – Eternal
54. Maan – Benevolence
55. Naim – Comfort, Tranquility
56. Osama – Lion
57. Qusay – Distant
58. Rashid – Rightly guided
59. Suhail – Canopus star
60. Tamim – Complete, Perfect
61. Walid – Newborn
62. Yaqub – Supplanter
63. Zakariya – God remembers
64. Ammar – Long-lived
65. Bilal – Water, Moisture
66. Fahim – Understanding
67. Hamid – Praiseworthy
68. Ilyas – The Lord is my God
69. Jibril – God is my strength

70. Khalil – Friend
71. Mahir – Skilled
72. Nawaf – High, Lofty
73. Othman – Baby bustard
74. Ra'ed – Leader
75. Saad – Good luck
76. Taha – Pure
77. Wajih – Distinguished
78. Youssef – He will add
79. Zuhair – Bright, Shining
80. Anas – Affection, Love
81. Badr – Full moon
82. Fawaz – Successful
83. Hashim – Destroyer of evil
84. Isa – Jesus
85. Jihad – Struggle
86. Khaled – Eternal
87. Majeed – Glorious
88. Nader – Rare
89. Omar – Life
90. Rafiq – Gentle, Friend
91. Sabir – Patient
92. Tawfiq – Success, Reconciliation
93. Waseem – Handsome
94. Yaqeen – Certainty
95. Ziad – Abundance
96. Aqil – Intelligent
97. Baha – Beautiful, Magnificent
98. Farouk – One who distinguishes truth from falsehood
99. Hasan – Handsome, Good
100. Izzat – Honor, Prestige

Syrian baby boy names

1. Ahmad - Highly praised or one who constantly thanks God
2. Bahij - Splendid, beautiful
3. Bashar - Bringer of good news
4. Dabir - Secretary or teacher
5. Elias - The Lord is my God
6. Fadi - Savior
7. Ghassan - Youth, prime of life
8. Hafez - Guardian, protector
9. Ihab - Gift
10. Jamil - Beautiful
11. Kadar - Powerful
12. Labib - Sensible, intelligent
13. Mahir - Skilled
14. Nizar - Little
15. Omar - Long-lived
16. Qasim - One who distributes
17. Rami - Archer
18. Samir - Entertaining companion
19. Tariq - Morning star
20. Umar - Flourishing, thriving
21. Walid - Newborn
22. Yasin - Rich, the name of a surah in the Quran
23. Ziad - Abundance
24. Adnan - Settler
25. Bilal - The chosen one
26. Chafik - Sympathizing
27. Daoud - Beloved
28. Emir - Prince, ruler
29. Fares - Knight
30. Ghiyath - Succorer
31. Hani - Happy, delighted
32. Ilyas - The Lord is my God

33. Jalal - Majesty
34. Kamal - Perfection
35. Latif - Gentle, kind
36. Majid - Noble, glorious
37. Nabil - Noble, generous
38. Qadir - Capable, powerful
39. Rafiq - Kind, friend
40. Sabir - Patient
41. Tawfik - Success, reconciliation
42. Uthman - Baby bustard
43. Wasim - Handsome, graceful
44. Yahya - God is gracious
45. Zuhair - Little flower
46. Adel - Just, fair
47. Bassam - Smiling
48. Chadi - Consoling
49. Dawood - Beloved, a Prophet's name
50. Essam - Safeguard
51. Farid - Unique
52. Ghaleb - Conqueror
53. Habib - Beloved
54. Ibrahim - Father of a multitude
55. Jalil - Great, revered
56. Karim - Generous, noble
57. Luqman - Wise
58. Majeed - Glorious
59. Nadeem - Companion, friend
60. Qais - Firm
61. Raed - Leader
62. Saad - Good luck
63. Taha - Pure
64. Usama - Lion
65. Wael - Seeker of refuge
66. Youssef - God will increase
67. Zain - Beauty, grace
68. Amjad - More glorious

69. Bilal - Moisture
70. Chawki - Pleasant
71. Diya - Light, glow
72. Eyad - Support, might, strength
73. Fawaz - Successful
74. Ghazi - Warrior
75. Hamza - Lion
76. Imad - Support, pillar
77. Jafar - Little stream
78. Khalid - Eternal, immortal
79. Laith - Lion
80. Marwan - Solid
81. Naseem - Breeze
82. Qusay - Distant
83. Rakan - Noble
84. Salim - Safe, sound
85. Talal - Nice, admirable
86. Uthman - Companion of the Prophet
87. Wajih - Noble
88. Yaqub - Supplanter
89. Zaid - Increase, growth
90. Anas - Affection, love
91. Bishr - Joy, happiness
92. Charbel - Story of God
93. Duraid - Old Arabic name
94. Ezzat - Respect, honor
95. Fahd - Lynx
96. Ghassan - Old Arabic name
97. Hamad - Praised
98. Ihsan - Beneficence
99. Jad - Generosity
100. Khalil - Friend

Lebanese baby boy names

1. Adnan - Settler, long-term resident
2. Ahmad - Praiseworthy, commendable
3. Akram - Most generous
4. Ali - Exalted, noble
5. Amin - Trustworthy, faithful
6. Amir - Prince, commander
7. Asad - Lion
8. Ayman - Lucky, on the right
9. Bashir - Bringer of good news
10. Basim - Smiling
11. Bilal - Water, freshness
12. Daoud - Beloved
13. Elias - The Lord is my God
14. Fadi - Redeemer, savior
15. Farid - Unique, singular
16. Faisal - Decisive, resolute
17. Ghassan - Youth, prime of life
18. Habib - Beloved, darling
19. Hadi - Guide to righteousness
20. Hamza - Strong, steadfast
21. Hasan - Handsome, good
22. Hisham - Generous, noble
23. Idris - Interpreter, studious
24. Imad - Pillar, support
25. Ismail - God will hear
26. Jamal - Beauty
27. Jamil - Beautiful
28. Jihad - Struggle, holy war
29. Kahlil - Friend
30. Kamal - Perfection, completeness
31. Karim - Generous, noble
32. Khalid - Eternal, immortal
33. Khaled - Eternal

34. Lutfi - Kind, gentle
35. Majd - Glory, honor
36. Majid - Glorious
37. Malik - King, owner
38. Marwan - Solid, quartz
39. Moe - Saved by God
40. Mohamad - The praised one
41. Moussa - Drawn out of the water
42. Nabil - Noble, generous
43. Nader - Rare, unique
44. Nadim - Drinking companion
45. Nasir - Helper, supporter
46. Omar - Flourishing, long-lived
47. Osman - Servant of God
48. Qasim - Divider, distributor
49. Rafiq - Gentle, kind
50. Raouf - Merciful, compassionate
51. Rashad - Rightly guided
52. Rida - Contentment, satisfaction
53. Rami - Archer
54. Riad - Gardens, meadows
55. Sabir - Patient
56. Saad - Happiness, luck
57. Saif - Sword
58. Salim - Safe, sound
59. Sami - High, exalted
60. Samir - Entertaining companion
61. Sharif - Noble, honorable
62. Tariq - Morning star
63. Walid - Newborn
64. Yasin - Prophet's name
65. Youssef - God will add
66. Ziad - Growth, abundance
67. Ziyad - To increase, growth
68. Zuhair - Little flower
69. Abbas - Stern, lion

70. Abdullah - Servant of God
71. Adel - Just, fair
72. Akeem - Wise, intelligent
73. Aziz - Powerful, beloved
74. Badr - Full moon
75. Bahir - Dazzling, brilliant
76. Fares - Knight
77. Galal - Greatness, pride
78. Hafez - Protector
79. Hakim - Wise, judicious
80. Halim - Gentle, patient
81. Harun - Exalted, noble
82. Haytham - Young eagle
83. Hussein - Handsome, beautiful
84. Ihab - Gift
85. Ihsan - Beneficence, charity
86. Ilyas - The Lord is my God
87. Imran - Prosperity, exalted nation
88. Iqbal - Prosperity, good fortune
89. Isa - God is salvation
90. Iskandar - Defender of mankind
91. Jad - Generous
92. Jahid - Industrious, hardworking
93. Jibril - God is my strength
94. Kareem - Noble, generous
95. Labib - Sensible, intelligent
96. Latif - Kind, gentle
97. Mahir - Skilled, expert
98. Mahmud - Praiseworthy
99. Muhannad - Sword
100. Mustafa - Chosen, selected

Kuwaiti baby boy names

1. Abdullah - Servant of God
2. Abdulrahman - Servant of the merciful one
3. Ahmed - Highly praised or one who constantly thanks God
4. Ali - Exalted, noble
5. Amir - Prince, commander
6. Ayman - Blessed, lucky
7. Bashar - Bringer of good news
8. Bilal - Refreshing, satisfying
9. Daoud - Beloved
10. Ebrahim - Father of many nations
11. Fahad - Leopard
12. Faris - Horseman, knight
13. Faisal - Decisive
14. Ghassan - Youth, prime of life
15. Habib - Beloved
16. Hamad - Praiseworthy
17. Hasan - Handsome, good
18. Husain - Handsome, beautiful
19. Ibrahim - Father of a multitude
20. Idris - Studious, knowledgeable
21. Imran - Prosperity, happiness
22. Isa - God is salvation
23. Jamal - Beauty, grace
24. Jassim - Great, big
25. Khaled - Eternal
26. Khalil - Friend
27. Majid - Glorious
28. Malik - King, owner
29. Mansoor - Victorious
30. Mohammed - Praised
31. Mubarak - Blessed
32. Mustafa - Chosen one

33. Nabeel - Noble, generous
34. Nader - Rare, unique
35. Omar - Long-lived
36. Qasim - Divider, distributor
37. Raed - Leader
38. Rashid - Rightly guided
39. Saad - Good luck
40. Saif - Sword
41. Saleh - Righteous
42. Salman - Safe
43. Sami - High, elevated
44. Tariq - Morning star
45. Waleed - Newborn
46. Yasser - Wealth, ease
47. Yasir - Wealthy
48. Yousef - God will increase
49. Zaid - Abundance, growth
50. Zain - Beauty, grace
51. Adel - Just, fair
52. Akeem - Wise, intelligent
53. Akram - Generous
54. Anas - Affection, love
55. Asad - Lion
56. Aziz - Powerful, beloved
57. Badr - Full moon
58. Basim - Smiling
59. Dhari - Fast
60. Emad - Pillar, support
61. Fadi - Redeemer, savior
62. Fawaz - Successful
63. Hadi - Guide
64. Hakim - Wise, judicious
65. Ihab - Gift
66. Ihsan - Beneficence, charity
67. Jalal - Majesty, glory
68. Kamal - Perfection, excellence

69. Karim - Generous, noble
70. Lutfi - Kind, gentle
71. Mahdi - Guided one
72. Majed - Noble, glorious
73. Moeen - Helper, supporter
74. Naim - Comfort, tranquility
75. Nawaf - High, lofty
76. Qais - Firm
77. Rafiq - Friend, companion
78. Ramzi - Symbolic
79. Sabir - Patient
80. Safwan - Rock
81. Suhail - Easy, uncomplicated
82. Taha - Pure
83. Talal - Admirable, nice
84. Tamim - Complete, perfect
85. Thamer - Fruitful, productive
86. Umar - Life, long living
87. Usama - Lion
88. Wael - Seeking shelter
89. Yaqub - Supplanter
90. Yasin - Prophet's name
91. Zakariya - God has remembered
92. Ziyad - Growth, abundance
93. Rami - Archer
94. Samir - Entertaining companion
95. Sufyan - Fast walker
96. Tawfiq - Success, reconciliation
97. Wahid - Unique, singular
98. Yahya - God is gracious
99. Zuhair - Bright, shining
100. Haris - Guardian, protector

Emirati baby boy names

1. Abdullah - Servant of God
2. Ahmed - Highly praised
3. Ali - Exalted, noble
4. Amir - Prince, ruler
5. Arif - Knowledgeable, wise
6. Ayman - Lucky, right-handed
7. Aziz - Powerful, respected
8. Badr - Full moon
9. Bilal - Water, moisture
10. Daoud - Beloved
11. Essam - Safeguard
12. Faisal - Decisive, judge
13. Faris - Horseman, knight
14. Ghassan - Youth, prime of life
15. Habib - Beloved, dear
16. Hadi - Guide to righteousness
17. Hamid - Praiseworthy
18. Haris - Guardian, protector
19. Ibrahim - Father of many
20. Idris - Studious, learned
21. Imran - Prosperity, happiness
22. Ismail - God will hear
23. Jamal - Beauty
24. Javed - Eternal, everlasting
25. Kadar - Powerful
26. Khalid - Eternal, immortal
27. Latif - Gentle, kind
28. Mahmoud - Praised
29. Mansoor - Victorious
30. Nabil - Noble, high-born
31. Omar - Long-lived
32. Qasim - Divider, distributor
33. Rashid - Rightly guided

34. Saad - Good luck
35. Sabir - Patient
36. Taha - Pure
37. Talib - Seeker, student
38. Umar - Life, long living
39. Waleed - Newborn
40. Yasin - The opening letters of Surah 36 in the Qur'an
41. Zahir - Bright, shining
42. Zayed - Growth, increase
43. Aamir - Full, prosperous
44. Bahir - Dazzling, brilliant
45. Basim - Smiling
46. Danyal - Intelligent
47. Ehsan - Charitable
48. Fahim - Understanding, intelligent
49. Ghalib - Victorious
50. Hakim - Wise, judicious
51. Iqbal - Prosperity, good fortune
52. Jafar - Stream
53. Kamal - Perfection
54. Lutfi - Kind, gentle
55. Muneer - Brilliant, shining
56. Naseer - Helper, protector
57. Qadir - Capable, powerful
58. Rafeeq - Gentle, kind
59. Samir - Entertaining companion
60. Tariq - Morning star
61. Ubaid - Servant of God
62. Wasi - Broad-minded
63. Yasir - Wealthy
64. Zafar - Victory
65. Adil - Just, fair
66. Bari - Creator
67. Dawood - Beloved
68. Emir - Commander, prince
69. Fadi - Redeemer, savior

70. Ghazi - Warrior
71. Hakeem - Wise
72. Irfan - Knowledge, learning
73. Jalal - Majesty, glory
74. Kareem - Generous, noble
75. Luqman - Wise
76. Mujeeb - Responsive
77. Nasir - Helper, supporter
78. Qayyum - Self-sustaining
79. Rafiq - Companion, friend
80. Sajid - One who prostrates
81. Tawfiq - Success, reconciliation
82. Ubayy - Servant of God
83. Wajid - Finder, affluent
84. Yaqub - Supplanter
85. Zaheer - Supporter, ally
86. Adnan - Settler
87. Bilal - Refreshing
88. Daud - Beloved
89. Fakhr - Pride, glory
90. Ghulam - Servant, boy
91. Hamza - Lion
92. Isa - Jesus
93. Jalil - Great, revered
94. Khaled - Eternal
95. Malik - King, owner
96. Nuh - Comfort, repose
97. Rafi - Exalted, sublime
98. Suhail - Easy, uncomplicated
99. Tariq - Morning star
100. Yusuf - He will add

Qatari baby boy names

1. Abdul - Servant of God
2. Ahmed - Praiseworthy
3. Ali - Exalted, Noble
4. Aamir - Prosperous
5. Bilal - Water, Moisture
6. Basim - Smiling
7. Bashar - Bringer of Good News
8. Badr - Full Moon
9. Daoud - Beloved
10. Faisal - Decisive
11. Faris - Knight, Horseman
12. Fahad - Leopard
13. Ghazi - Conqueror
14. Hamad - Praiseworthy
15. Hassan - Handsome, Good
16. Hadi - Guide to Righteousness
17. Ibrahim - Father of Many
18. Imran - Prosperity
19. Jamal - Beauty
20. Jassim - Great, Big
21. Khaled - Eternal
22. Khalil - Friend
23. Karim - Generous
24. Latif - Gentle, Kind
25. Majid - Noble, Glorious
26. Mohammed - Praiseworthy
27. Mansoor - Victorious
28. Nabeel - Noble
29. Nasser - Helper, Supporter
30. Omar - Long-lived
31. Osman - Servant of God
32. Qasim - Divider
33. Rashid - Rightly Guided

34. Saad - Good Luck
35. Saleh - Righteous
36. Tariq - Morning Star
37. Uthman - Companion of Prophet
38. Waleed - Newborn
39. Youssef - God will Increase
40. Zaid - Abundance
41. Zahir - Bright, Shining
42. Adel - Just, Fair
43. Aziz - Powerful, Beloved
44. Barak - Blessing
45. Dinar - Gold Coin
46. Emir - Prince, Commander
47. Fadi - Savior
48. Ghalib - Victor
49. Habib - Beloved
50. Idris - Studious
51. Jafar - Stream
52. Kamil - Perfect
53. Lutfi - Kind, Gentle
54. Mubarak - Blessed
55. Nasir - Helper, Protector
56. Rafiq - Friend, Gentle
57. Sabir - Patient
58. Tawfiq - Success, Reconciliation
59. Yasir - Wealthy
60. Zahid - Ascetic, Devout
61. Ammar - Long-lived
62. Bahir - Dazzling, Brilliant
63. Daud - Beloved
64. Essam - Safeguard
65. Farhan - Happy, Joyful
66. Ghassan - Youth, Prime of Life
67. Hakim - Wise, Judge
68. Ilyas - The Lord is my God
69. Jibril - God is my Strength

70. Kamal - Perfection
71. Luqman - Wise
72. Mustafa - Chosen One
73. Naim - Comfort, Tranquility
74. Raheem - Merciful
75. Samir - Entertaining Companion
76. Talal - Admirable
77. Yaqub - Supplanter
78. Zaki - Pure
79. Aqil - Intelligent
80. Bashar - Bringer of Good Tidings
81. Dhiya - Light, Splendor
82. Fakhr - Pride, Glory
83. Ghayth - Rain
84. Hisham - Generous
85. Ismail - God will Hear
86. Jalal - Majesty, Glory
87. Khair - Goodness, Welfare
88. Layth - Lion
89. Mufid - Useful
90. Nawaf - High, Lofty
91. Rafid - Supporter
92. Saif - Sword
93. Taha - Pure
94. Yahya - God is Gracious
95. Zuhair - Little Flower
96. Asim - Protector, Guardian
97. Baha - Beautiful, Magnificent
98. Dhul - Possessor
99. Fawaz - Successful
100. Ghulam - Servant, Boy

Omani baby boy names

1. Abdullah - Servant of God
2. Abdulrahman - Servant of the Merciful
3. Ahmed - Highly praised or one who constantly thanks God
4. Ali - Exalted, noble
5. Ameer - Prince, ruler
6. Badr - Full moon
7. Bilal - Water, moisture, freshness
8. Fahad - Leopard, lynx
9. Faisal - Decisive, arbiter
10. Faris - Horseman, knight
11. Ghassan - Youth, prime of life
12. Hamad - Praiseworthy
13. Hassan - Beautiful, handsome
14. Ibrahim - Father of multitude
15. Idris - Studious, knowledgeable
16. Imran - Prosperity, happiness
17. Issa - God is salvation
18. Jamal - Beauty
19. Jasim - Great, big, huge
20. Kadar - Powerful
21. Khalid - Eternal, immortal
22. Majid - Noble, glorious
23. Malik - King, owner
24. Mohammed - Praised, commendable
25. Nasser - Helper, supporter
26. Omar - Flourishing, long-lived
27. Qasim - One who distributes
28. Rashid - Rightly guided
29. Saif - Sword
30. Salman - Safe, whole, flawless
31. Tariq - Morning star
32. Yahya - God is gracious

33. Zakaria - God remembers
34. Zayed - To increase, growth
35. Aban - Clear, lucid
36. Adnan - Settler
37. Afnan - Branches of a tree
38. Aqil - Intelligent, wise
39. Ayman - Blessed, lucky
40. Baha - Beautiful, magnificent
41. Basim - Smiling
42. Daud - Beloved
43. Emir - Prince, commander
44. Fadi - Redeemer, savior
45. Ghalib - Conqueror
46. Hakim - Wise, judicious
47. Ilyas - The Lord is my God
48. Jabir - Comforter, bringer of consolation
49. Karim - Generous, noble
50. Latif - Gentle, kind
51. Madani - Civilized
52. Nabil - Noble, high born
53. Othman - Companion of the Prophet
54. Qadir - Capable, powerful
55. Rafiq - Gentle, friend
56. Sabir - Patient
57. Talib - Seeker, student
58. Ubaid - Small slave
59. Waleed - Newborn
60. Yasin - Prophet's name
61. Zahir - Bright, shining
62. Abbad - Worshipper of God
63. Adil - Just, honest
64. Ahsan - The best of all
65. Akram - More generous
66. Ayub - Prophet's name, Job
67. Bilal - The first Muezzin
68. Da'wud - Beloved; a Prophet's name

69. Ehab - Gift
70. Fakhr - Pride, glory
71. Ghazi - Warrior
72. Habib - Beloved
73. Irfan - Gratefulness
74. Jafar - Stream
75. Khalil - Friend
76. Latif - Kind, gentle
77. Mahir - Skilled
78. Naim - Comfort, tranquility
79. Osama - Lion
80. Qais - Firm
81. Ra'id - Leader
82. Sadiq - Truthful
83. Taha - A chapter of the Quran
84. Umar - Life, long living
85. Wajih - Noble
86. Yasir - Wealthy
87. Zain - Beautiful, handsome
88. Abbas - Stern, lion
89. Adham - Black
90. Ahmad - Much praised
91. Ammar - Long-lived
92. Bahir - Dazzling, brilliant
93. Bassam - Smiling
94. Dawood - Beloved, a Prophet's name
95. Fadi - Savior
96. Ghayth - Rain
97. Haris - Guardian, protector
98. Ismail - God will hear
99. Jalal - Glory
100. Kamal - Perfection

Bahraini baby boy names

1. Abdul - servant of God
2. Ahmed - praiseworthy
3. Ali - exalted or noble
4. Amir - prince
5. Ayman - blessed or lucky
6. Bashar - bringer of good news
7. Bilal - water or moisture
8. Daoud - beloved or dear
9. Ebrahim - father of many
10. Faisal - decisive
11. Faizan - grace or charity
12. Ghassan - youth or prime of life
13. Hadi - guide to righteousness
14. Hamza - strong or steadfast
15. Hassan - handsome or good
16. Imran - exalted nation
17. Ishaq - laughter
18. Jamal - beauty
19. Khaled - eternal
20. Khalil - friend
21. Latif - kind or gentle
22. Malik - king or owner
23. Mansoor - victorious
24. Mubarak - blessed
25. Nabil - noble or generous
26. Omar - flourishing or long-lived
27. Qasim - one who distributes
28. Rafiq - kind or gentle
29. Rashid - rightly guided
30. Saad - luck or good fortune
31. Sameer - entertaining companion
32. Tariq - morning star
33. Usman - baby bustard

34. Waleed - newborn
35. Yahya - God is gracious
36. Yousif - God will increase
37. Zafar - victory
38. Zain - beauty or grace
39. Haris - guardian or protector
40. Idris - interpreter
41. Jafar - stream
42. Karim - generous
43. Luqman - wise
44. Majid - glorious
45. Nasir - helper or protector
46. Qadir - capable or powerful
47. Rami - archer
48. Sami - elevated or sublime
49. Taha - A name of Prophet Muhammad
50. Ubaid - small slave
51. Zahid - ascetic
52. Akram - most generous
53. Basim - one who smiles
54. Fadil - generous
55. Ghalib - victor
56. Hakim - wise or judicious
57. Ilyas - the Lord is my God
58. Jawad - generous
59. Khalid - immortal
60. Latif - gentle or kind
61. Munir - luminous or radiant
62. Nizar - little
63. Qasim - one who distributes
64. Raed - leader
65. Safwan - rock
66. Tawfiq - success or reconciliation
67. Umar - life
68. Walid - newborn
69. Ya'qub - supplanter

70. Yusuf - God will add
71. Zahir - bright or shining
72. Adnan - settler
73. Bilal - water or moisture
74. Daud - beloved
75. Fahad - panther or leopard
76. Ghazi - warrior
77. Habib - beloved
78. Imad - pillar or support
79. Jalal - greatness
80. Kamal - perfection
81. Layth - lion
82. Majid - noble
83. Naim - comfort or tranquility
84. Qadir - capable
85. Rashad - right guidance
86. Sabir - patient
87. Tariq - morning star
88. Uthman - baby bustard
89. Wajid - finder or inventor
90. Yasin - A chapter in the Quran
91. Zaki - pure
92. Adel - righteous
93. Badr - full moon
94. Dhiya - light or splendor
95. Farid - unique
96. Ghulam - servant or boy
97. Hakim - wise
98. Irfan - knowledge or awareness
99. Javed - eternal
100. Kamran - successful

Pakistani baby boy names

1. Aaban – Name of the angel
2. Aabid – Worshipper
3. Aahil – Prince
4. Aarib – Handsome, healthy
5. Aarif – Knowing, aware
6. Aariz – Respectable man
7. Aasim – Person who refrains from doing evil
8. Aayan – God's gift
9. Aazim – Determined
10. Abbas – Lion
11. Abdal – Servant of Allah
12. Abdul – Servant of God
13. Adil – Just, honest
14. Adnan – Settler
15. Afaq – The place where the Earth and Sky meet
16. Afraz – Standing tall like a mountain
17. Ahmad – Highly praised, commendable
18. Ahsan – The best of all
19. Ajmal – More beautiful
20. Akbar – Great
21. Akmal – Perfect, complete
22. Alam – World, universe
23. Ali – Exalted, noble
24. Altaf – Kindness
25. Amaan – Peace, protection
26. Ameer – Commander, prince
27. Amir – Prince, ruler
28. Anas – Affection, love
29. Anwar – Light
30. Arham – Mercy, compassion
31. Asad – Lion
32. Asif – Gather, harvest
33. Atif – Kind, sympathetic

34. Ayaan – Gift of God
35. Aziz – Powerful, respected
36. Babar – Lion, king of jungle
37. Badar – Full moon
38. Bahadur – Brave, courageous
39. Basir – One who sees
40. Bilal – The first muezzin (caller to prayer)
41. Burhan – Proof, evidence
42. Daanish – Wisdom, learning
43. Dawood – Beloved friend
44. Ehsan – Charitable, compassionate
45. Faiz – Super abundance, effluence
46. Faraz – Elevation
47. Farhan – Joyful, happy
48. Faisal – Decisive, judge
49. Farid – Unique, matchless
50. Feroz – Successful
51. Ghazi – Conqueror
52. Hadi – Guide to righteousness
53. Hamza – Lion, strong
54. Haris – Guardian, protector
55. Hasan – Handsome, good
56. Hashim – Destroyer of evil
57. Hussain – Handsome, beautiful
58. Ibrahim – Father of multitude
59. Idris – Studious person
60. Imran – Prosperity, happiness
61. Iqbal – Prosperity, good fortune
62. Irfan – Thankfulness
63. Ismail – God will hear
64. Jahangir – World conqueror
65. Jamal – Beauty
66. Jawad – Generous, noble
67. Kamal – Perfection, excellence
68. Kashif – Revealer of secrets
69. Khalid – Eternal, immortal

70. Khurram – Delighted, joyful
71. Latif – Gentle, kind
72. Maaz – Brave man
73. Mahir – Skilled, expert
74. Majid – Noble, glorious
75. Mansoor – Victorious, triumphant
76. Moiz – Respectful, one who gives protection
77. Mustafa – Chosen one
78. Nabeel – Noble man
79. Nadeem – Companion, friend
80. Nasir – Helper, protector
81. Omar – Life, long living
82. Osman – Tender youth
83. Qasim – One who distributes
84. Raheem – Merciful
85. Rahman – Compassionate
86. Rashid – Rightly guided
87. Raza – Consent, satisfaction
88. Rehan – Scented, blessing from God
89. Saad – Good luck
90. Saif – Sword
91. Salman – Safe, mild, affable
92. Sami – Elevated, sublime
93. Shahid – Witness
94. Shoaib – Who shows the right path
95. Taha – Pure
96. Talha – Kind of tree
97. Tariq – Morning star
98. Usman – The young of a lark, a beautiful pen, name of the third Caliph of Islam
99. Waleed – Newborn child
100. Zain – Beauty, grace

Bangladeshi baby boy names

1. Aahil - Prince
2. Aariz - Respectable
3. Aayan - Gift of God
4. Abir - Colorful
5. Adnan - Settler
6. Ahsan - Compassionate
7. Ahyan - Gift of God
8. Aizaz - Respect
9. Amaan - Peace
10. Arham - Merciful
11. Asif - Gather
12. Ayman - Lucky
13. Azan - Call for prayer
14. Bari - Creator
15. Basit - Vast
16. Bilal - Water
17. Burhan - Proof
18. Daanish - Wisdom
19. Ehan - Full moon
20. Fahad - Lynx
21. Faizan - Beneficence
22. Farhan - Happy
23. Faisal - Judge
24. Faysal - Decisive
25. Ghazi - Warrior
26. Hadi - Guide to righteousness
27. Hamza - Lion
28. Haris - Guardian
29. Hasan - Handsome
30. Hashim - Destroyer of evil
31. Hussain - Handsome
32. Ibrahim - Father of a multitude
33. Idris - Studious

34. Imran - Prosperity
35. Irfan - Gratefulness
36. Ismail - God will hear
37. Jafar - Rivulet
38. Jamal - Beauty
39. Junaid - Soldier
40. Kamal - Perfection
41. Karim - Generous
42. Khalid - Eternal
43. Khurram - Cheerful
44. Latif - Kind
45. Maaz - Brave man
46. Mahir - Skilled
47. Majid - Noble
48. Mansoor - Victorious
49. Masood - Happy
50. Mirza - Prince
51. Mubarak - Blessed
52. Mustafa - The chosen one
53. Nabeel - Noble
54. Nadeem - Friend
55. Nafiz - Influential
56. Omar - Flourishing, long-lived
57. Osman - Tender youth
58. Qasim - Divider
59. Rafiq - Friend
60. Rahim - Merciful
61. Rahman - Merciful
62. Raheel - One who shows the way
63. Rais - Captain
64. Rashid - Rightly guided
65. Rayhan - Fragrant
66. Rehan - Scented
67. Saad - Good luck
68. Sabir - Patient
69. Salman - Safe

70. Sami - High, exalted
71. Shafiq - Compassionate
72. Shahid - Witness
73. Shams - Sun
74. Sharif - Noble
75. Sohail - Moonlight
76. Taha - Pure
77. Taimur - Iron
78. Talha - Kind of tree
79. Tanvir - Enlightened
80. Tariq - Morning star
81. Umar - Life
82. Usman - The young of a bird
83. Wahid - Unique
84. Wasi - Broad-minded
85. Yasir - Wealthy
86. Yasin - Prophet's name
87. Yousuf - God will add
88. Zafar - Victory
89. Zahir - Bright, shining
90. Zain - Beauty
91. Zakir - Remembering
92. Zaman - Time, era
93. Zayed - Growth
94. Zia - Light
95. Zohair - Best friend of the last prophet
96. Zubair - Strong, firm
97. Azaan - Call for prayer
98. Saiful - Sword of
99. Arif - Knowledgeable
100. Raqib - Observer

Sri Lankan baby boy names

1. Abhaya – Fearless
2. Achala – Immovable
3. Adithya – Sun
4. Amila – Immeasurable
5. Amith – Friend
6. Ananda – Happiness
7. Anoj – Clear
8. Aravinda – Lotus
9. Aruna – Sun
10. Asanka – Without doubt
11. Ashen – King of wish
12. Asiri – Blessings
13. Bandara – Leader
14. Bimal – Pure
15. Chamara – Helper
16. Chamindu – Bright
17. Charana – Foot
18. Chatura – Clever
19. Danuka – Bright morning
20. Dasun – Servant of God
21. Dayan – Merciful
22. Deepal – Light
23. Devinda – God of gods
24. Dhanushka – Bow
25. Dinuka – Bright day
26. Dulan – Heart
27. Erantha – Unique
28. Gavesh – Seeker
29. Harinda – Golden
30. Harsha – Happiness
31. Hasith – Happy
32. Heshan – God of satisfaction
33. Indika – Bright drop

34. Isuru – Radiant
35. Janith – Born
36. Jayasanka – Victorious
37. Kavinda – Poet
38. Keshan – Light of God
39. Kusal – Clever
40. Lakshan – Distinguished
41. Lasith – Brightness
42. Madhawa – Sweet like honey
43. Mahanama – Great name
44. Malinda – Dark
45. Manuka – Human
46. Methun – Friend
47. Nalin – Lotus
48. Nandana – Son
49. Navindu – New moon
50. Nimna – Excellent
51. Ovin – Bird
52. Pahan – Light
53. Pramuka – Chief
54. Prasad – Blessing
55. Raveen – Sun
56. Roshan – Bright
57. Sachin – Pure existence
58. Sadun – Good heart
59. Saman – Equal
60. Sanuka – Bright
61. Sathuka – Truthful
62. Senura – Golden radiance
63. Shalinda – Protecting
64. Shihan – Teacher
65. Sujan – Honest
66. Supun – Dream
67. Tharindu – Moon
68. Uvin – Light
69. Vihanga – Bird

70. Yasas – Fame
71. Yohan – God is gracious
72. Yuvan – Young
73. Zayan – Bright
74. Thamindu – Bright moon
75. Ishan – Sun
76. Kaveen – Beautiful
77. Lahiru – Sun
78. Madushan – Sweet person
79. Navod – New
80. Pasindu – Shining
81. Ruvin – God of beauty
82. Sahan – Patience
83. Thenuka – Intelligent
84. Udara – Noble
85. Vimukthi – Freedom
86. Yasith – Successful
87. Buddhika – Enlightened one
88. Chathura – Brilliant
89. Dineth – Sun
90. Harindu – Golden
91. Isuranga – King of beauty
92. Januka – Son
93. Kasun – Ray of light
94. Lashan – Brightness
95. Maduranga – Sweet color
96. Naveen – New
97. Osanda – Immortal
98. Praveen – Skilled
99. Rukshan – Bright
100. Samith – Friendly

Nepali baby boy names

1. Aadesh – Command
2. Aarav – Peaceful
3. Abhinav – New
4. Aditya – Sun
5. Aman – Peace
6. Amit – Infinite
7. Anish – Supreme
8. Arjun – Bright, Shining
9. Ashok – Without sorrow
10. Avinash – Indestructible
11. Bimal – Pure
12. Bishal – Great
13. Chandra – Moon
14. Deepak – Lamp, Light
15. Dinesh – Sun
16. Gagan – Sky
17. Gautam – Bright
18. Hari – God Vishnu
19. Ishan – Sun
20. Jeevan – Life
21. Keshav – Another name for Lord Krishna
22. Krishna – Dark, Black
23. Lokesh – King of the world
24. Madan – God of Love
25. Manish – God of Mind
26. Mohan – Charming
27. Nabin – New
28. Niranjan – Pure
29. Omkar – The sound of the sacred syllable
30. Prakash – Light
31. Rajan – King
32. Ramesh – Lord of Rama
33. Roshan – Bright, Shining

34. Sagar – Ocean
35. Suman – Flower
36. Suraj – Sun
37. Utsav – Festival
38. Vishnu – Preserver of the universe
39. Yash – Glory, Fame
40. Aakarshan – Attraction
41. Bhaskar – Sun
42. Chandan – Sandalwood
43. Dhiraj – Patience
44. Eklavya – Student who learned bow by himself
45. Gyanendra – Lord of Knowledge
46. Harshit – Happy
47. Indra – King of Gods
48. Jagdish – Lord of the World
49. Kapil – Fair
50. Laxman – Brother of Lord Rama
51. Mahesh – Great Ruler
52. Naveen – New
53. Pranav – Sacred syllable Om
54. Rishabh – Superior
55. Samar – Battle, Conflict
56. Tanmay – Engrossed
57. Ujjwal – Bright, Clear
58. Vimal – Clean, Pure
59. Yuvraj – Prince
60. Aarush – First rays of the sun
61. Bijay – Victory
62. Chetan – Consciousness
63. Devendra – King of Gods
64. Eshan – Lord Shiva
65. Hrithik – From the heart
66. Ishaan – Sun
67. Jayendra – Lord of victory
68. Keshab – Another name for Lord Krishna
69. Lalit – Beautiful

70. Mahendra – King
71. Nishant – Dawn
72. Pranesh – Lord of life
73. Rupesh – Lord of beauty
74. Sambhav – Possible
75. Tapan – Sun
76. Uday – To rise
77. Vivek – Wisdom
78. Yashpal – Protector of fame
79. Aayush – Long life
80. Brijesh – Lord of Brij land
81. Chirag – Lamp
82. Deepesh – Lord of light
83. Ekansh – Whole
84. Govinda – Lord Krishna
85. Harshad – Giver of joy
86. Indraneel – Emerald
87. Jagat – World
88. Kamal – Lotus
89. Loknath – Lord of the world
90. Manoj – Born of the mind
91. Naman – Salutation
92. Prabhat – Morning
93. Rajesh – King of Kings
94. Surya – Sun
95. Tarun – Young
96. Utkarsh – Progress
97. Vikas – Development
98. Yatin – Ascetic
99. Abhay – Fearless
100. Bijesh – Lord Shiva

Bhutanese baby boy names

1. Tashi - Prosperity
2. Choki - Peace
3. Jigme - Fearless
4. Dorji - Thunderbolt
5. Kuenzang - Universal Excellence
6. Phurba - Sky Iron
7. Pema - Lotus
8. Wangchuk - Conqueror
9. Chimi - Immortal
10. Dawa - Moon
11. Sonam - Merit
12. Lhendup - Growth
13. Tempa - Teachings of Buddha
14. Tshering - Long Life
15. Rinchen - Precious Gem
16. Gyeltshen - King's Victory
17. Karma - Action
18. Tenzin - Holder of Buddha's Teachings
19. Ugyen - Representative of Buddha
20. Gyem - Jewel
21. Tobgay - Upholder of Merit
22. Yonten - Knowledgeable
23. Sangay - Buddha
24. Phuntsho - Prosperity
25. Kinley - Benevolent
26. Jamyang - Gentle Voice
27. Namgyel - Victorious in All Directions
28. Norbu - Jewel
29. Sherab - Wisdom
30. Zangpo - Good
31. Damcho - Noble Lamp
32. Dechen - Great Happiness
33. Drakpa - Brave

34. Gawa - Joy
35. Jampa - Loving Kindness
36. Kencho - All-Knowing
37. Loday - Intelligent
38. Nidup - Restful
39. Om - Sacred Syllable in Buddhism
40. Paljor - Glorious
41. Rabsel - Clear Light
42. Sangpo - Kind
43. Tharchin - Upholder of the Teachings
44. Yeshey - Wisdom
45. Zopa - Patient
46. Chophel - Dharma Flourishing
47. Dorje - Indestructible
48. Gyurme - Everlasting
49. Jigten - Worldly
50. Kalsang - Good Fortune
51. Lhawang - Power
52. Migmar - Fire
53. Nyima - Sun
54. Palden - Glorious
55. Rigzin - Holder of the Lineage
56. Samdrup - Fulfillment of Wishes
57. Tsewang - Life Empowerment
58. Wangdi - Power
59. Yeshi - Wisdom
60. Zangmo - Good Woman
61. Choden - Religious
62. Druk - Dragon
63. Gyatso - Ocean
64. Jangchub - Enlightenment
65. Kunga - All Joy
66. Lhamo - Goddess
67. Namdak - Pure
68. Pema - Lotus
69. Rinpoche - Precious One

70. Samten - Meditation
71. Tashi - Auspicious
72. Wangmo - Queen
73. Yonten - Knowledge
74. Zopa - Patience
75. Chosang - Dharma Increase
76. Dorje - Diamond
77. Gyurmed - Long Life
78. Jampal - Gentle Glory
79. Karma - Action
80. Lhundup - Spontaneous
81. Migyur - Unchanging
82. Nima - Sun
83. Palmo - Glorious
84. Rigsel - Clear Light
85. Samdup - Aspiration
86. Tenzing - Upholder of Teachings
87. Wangchuk - Power
88. Yeshe - Wisdom
89. Zangpo - Good
90. Chokden - Supreme Dharma
91. Drukpa - Dragon
92. Gyurme - Infinite
93. Jampa - Love
94. Kunchen - All Knowing
95. Lhakpa - Wednesday
96. Namkha - Sky
97. Pelden - Glorious
98. Rinchen - Precious Gem
99. Samphel - Fulfillment of Wishes
100. Tashi - Prosperity

Afghan baby boy names

1. Abdullah – Servant of God
2. Adil – Fair, Honest
3. Ahmad – Highly Praised
4. Ali – Exalted, Noble
5. Aman – Security, Peace
6. Arif – Knowledgeable
7. Asad – Lion
8. Ashraf – Noble, Honorable
9. Atif – Compassionate, Affectionate
10. Babur – Tiger
11. Badr – Full Moon
12. Basir – One Who Sees
13. Bilal – Refreshing
14. Burhan – Proof
15. Daoud – Beloved
16. Ehsan – Charitable
17. Farid – Unique
18. Faisal – Decisive
19. Ghulam – Servant
20. Habib – Beloved
21. Hadi – Guide
22. Hamid – Praiseworthy
23. Harun – Exalted, Noble
24. Hasan – Handsome
25. Husayn – Beautiful
26. Ibrahim – Father of Many
27. Idris – Studious
28. Imran – Prosperity
29. Iqbal – Prosperity
30. Ismail – God will Hear
31. Jamal – Beauty
32. Jawad – Generous
33. Kabir – Great

34. Kamal – Perfection
35. Karim – Generous
36. Khalid – Eternal
37. Khurram – Delighted
38. Latif – Gentle, Kind
39. Majid – Noble
40. Malik – King
41. Mansur – Victorious
42. Masood – Lucky
43. Mustafa – Chosen One
44. Nadeem – Companion
45. Nasir – Helper
46. Naveed – Good News
47. Omar – Flourishing, Long Life
48. Qadir – Capable
49. Qasim – Divider
50. Rahim – Merciful
51. Rais – Captain
52. Rashid – Rightly Guided
53. Reza – Contentment
54. Saad – Good Fortune
55. Saeed – Happy
56. Salah – Righteousness
57. Sami – Elevated
58. Sarwar – Chief
59. Shafiq – Compassionate
60. Shah – King
61. Shakir – Thankful
62. Shams – Sun
63. Sharif – Noble
64. Siddiq – Truthful
65. Sohail – Gentle, Easy
66. Tahir – Pure
67. Talib – Seeker
68. Tariq – Morning Star
69. Umar – Life

70. Usman – The Young of a Bird
71. Waleed – Newborn Child
72. Wasim – Handsome
73. Yasin – Prophet's Name
74. Yousuf – God will Add
75. Zafar – Victory
76. Zahir – Shining, Luminous
77. Zain – Grace
78. Zaki – Pure
79. Zubair – Strong, Firm
80. Feroz – Successful
81. Jahangir – World Conqueror
82. Parvez – Success
83. Rahmat – Mercy
84. Suhail – Canopus Star
85. Taimur – Iron
86. Wahid – Unique
87. Yasir – Wealthy
88. Zakir – Remembering
89. Iftikhar – Pride
90. Mubarak – Blessed
91. Nusrat – Help, Aid
92. Qayyum – Self-Sustaining
93. Rizwan – Acceptance
94. Shuja – Brave
95. Tayyab – Pure
96. Uzair – Name of a Prophet
97. Waqar – Dignity, Sobriety
98. Yaqub – Supplanter
99. Zulfiqar – Cleaver of the Spine
100. Ilyas – The Lord is My God

Kazakhstani baby boy names

1. Abay – prudent
2. Adil – just
3. Aidar – moon
4. Akbar – great
5. Alikhan – noble prince
6. Almas – diamond
7. Altynbek – golden prince
8. Amangeldi – given by God
9. Amanzhol – peaceful path
10. Anuar – bright
11. Arman – desire
12. Aslan – lion
13. Askar – soldier
14. Azamat – greatness
15. Bagdat – name of a city in Iraq
16. Bakhytzhan – lucky soul
17. Baurzhan – rich soul
18. Bekzat – noble and independent
19. Berik – gift
20. Bolat – steel
21. Chingiz – name of the Mongolian conqueror
22. Daulet – wealth
23. Duman – fog
24. Edil – noble
25. Erasyl – noble
26. Erbolat – noble steel
27. Ermek – work
28. Galym – knowledge
29. Gani – rich
30. Ilyas – God is my Lord
31. Iskander – defender of mankind
32. Jaksylyk – goodness
33. Kairat – generosity

34. Kanat – wing
35. Kassym – divider
36. Kazybek – leader
37. Kenzhe – sage
38. Kuanysh – joy
39. Madina – city
40. Marat – desire for something
41. Meirzhan – charming soul
42. Mereke – celebration
43. Nurlan – baby falcon
44. Oraz – prosperous
45. Orken – horizon
46. Orynbek – prince of the universe
47. Rakhym – merciful
48. Ruslan – lion
49. Sabit – firm
50. Sagyndyk – beloved
51. Samat – independence
52. Serik – light
53. Shyngys – conqueror
54. Sultan – ruler
55. Tair – bird
56. Talgat – full moon
57. Tolegen – descendant of spirit
58. Ulan – warrior
59. Yerbol – given by the leader
60. Yerlan – baby falcon
61. Zhanbolat – soul of steel
62. Zhandos – soul of the universe
63. Zhasulan – bright boy
64. Zhumabek – prince of the people
65. Adyr – respect
66. Aibek – master of the moon
67. Aidos – shy
68. Aigul – moon flower
69. Aisultan – moon sultan

70. Aitzhan – soul of the moon
71. Akzhol – white path
72. Alibek – noble prince
73. Alimzhan – knowledgeable soul
74. Alpamys – name of a Kazakh folk hero
75. Altair – bird
76. Amanullah – peace of God
77. Amirkhan – prince
78. Arystan – lion
79. Asylbek – noble prince
80. Aybek – master of the moon
81. Aydin – enlightened
82. Aynur – moonlight
83. Azizbek – dear prince
84. Baibolat – rich steel
85. Baiterek – name of a monument in Kazakhstan
86. Batyr – hero
87. Beibarys – noble leopard
88. Beibit – peaceful
89. Bekbolat – noble steel
90. Beknur – noble light
91. Berikbol – gifted
92. Bolatbek – steel prince
93. Damir – heart
94. Daniar – knowledgeable
95. Dastan – story
96. Dias – light
97. Dinmukhamed – religion of Muhammad
98. Dosym – my love
99. Dulat – wealth
100. Erbol – leader

Uzbekistani baby boy names

1. Abdujalil – Servant of the Great
2. Abdujabbar – Servant of the Compeller
3. Abdukadir – Servant of the Capable
4. Abdumalik – Servant of the King
5. Abduvahid – Servant of the One
6. Abdurahim – Servant of the Merciful
7. Abdurashid – Servant of the Rightly Guided
8. Abdusami – Servant of the All Hearing
9. Abdusattor – Servant of the Creator
10. Abdushukur – Servant of the Thankful
11. Adham – Black
12. Akmal – Perfect
13. Alim – Knowledgeable
14. Alisher – Lion of God
15. Almas – Diamond
16. Anvar – Brighter
17. Asadbek – Lion Prince
18. Azamat – Greatness
19. Azim – Determined
20. Aziz – Dear
21. Babur – Lion
22. Bahodir – Brave
23. Bakhtiyor – Lucky
24. Bakhodir – Gift of God
25. Botir – Hero
26. Daler – Brave
27. Daniyar – Wise
28. Davron – Time
29. Dilshod – Happy Heart
30. Doniyor – Wealthy
31. Elyor – Superior
32. Erkin – Free
33. Farhod – Happy

34. Farrukh – Happy
35. Firdavs – Paradise
36. Furkat – Separation
37. G'ani – Rich
38. Hasan – Handsome
39. Husan – Beauty
40. Ibrohim – Father of Many
41. Ilhom – Inspiration
42. Islom – Submission to God
43. Jahongir – Conqueror of the World
44. Jalol – Greatness
45. Jamshid – Sun
46. Jasur – Brave
47. Javohir – Jewel
48. Javlon – Tall
49. Kamol – Perfection
50. Karim – Generous
51. Khurshid – Sun
52. Komil – Perfect
53. Maruf – Known
54. Mirzabek – Prince
55. Murod – Desire
56. Nodir – Rare
57. Nozim – Intention
58. O'ktam – Eighth
59. Odil – Justice
60. Olim – High
61. Orif – Knowledgeable
62. Otabek – Prince of the City
63. Ozodbek – Free Prince
64. Pulat – Steel
65. Qobil – Able
66. Qodir – Powerful
67. Qosim – Divider
68. Qurbon – Sacrifice
69. Rahmat – Mercy

70. Rashid – Rightly Guided
71. Ravshan – Bright
72. Rustam – Hero
73. Sabir – Patient
74. Said – Happy
75. Samandar – Ocean
76. Sarvar – Leader
77. Shams – Sun
78. Shavkat – Dignity
79. Sherzod – Lion's Son
80. Shohruh – Famous
81. Shukhrat – Glory
82. Shuhrat – Fame
83. Sirojiddin – Light of Religion
84. Sobir – Patient
85. Sodiq – Truthful
86. Sohib – Owner
87. Sulton – Sultan
88. Tohir – Pure
89. Umid – Hope
90. Utkir – Dig
91. Uzoq – Long
92. Valijon – Power
93. Xolmat – Generous
94. Xurshid – Sun
95. Yorqin – Bright
96. Zafar – Victory
97. Zahir – Bright
98. Ziyod – Increase
99. Zokir – Remember
100. Zohid – Ascetic

Tajikistani baby boy names

1. Abubakr – Noble, respected
2. Adham – Black
3. Aftab – The sun
4. Akmal – Perfect
5. Ali – Exalted
6. Alisher – Lion of God
7. Almas – Diamond
8. Amanullah – Trust of God
9. Anvar – Brighter
10. Arslan – Lion
11. Asadbek – Brave like a lion
12. Asif – Gatherer
13. Azamat – Majesty
14. Aziz – Powerful
15. Azizbek – Noble prince
16. Bahodur – Brave
17. Bakhtiyor – Lucky
18. Bahriddin – Sea of religion
19. Behruz – Good day
20. Bilol – Devoted to God
21. Bobur – Lion
22. Daler – Brave
23. Davlat – State
24. Dilshod – Happy heart
25. Fakhriddin – Pride of religion
26. Farhod – Happy
27. Farrukh – Happy, auspicious
28. Firdavs – Paradise
29. Firuz – Successful
30. Hasan – Handsome
31. Husan – Beauty
32. Ibrohim – Father of a multitude
33. Ilhom – Inspiration

34. Ismoil – God will hear
35. Jahongir – Conqueror of the world
36. Jaloliddin – Glory of religion
37. Jamol – Beauty
38. Jamshed – Sun
39. Javohir – Gem
40. Jovid – Eternal
41. Kambiz – Fortunate
42. Kamol – Perfection
43. Karim – Generous
44. Khurshed – Sun
45. Komil – Perfect
46. Madina – City of the Prophet
47. Mahmad – Praiseworthy
48. Mansur – Victorious
49. Mirzobek – Prince
50. Mubin – Clear, evident
51. Mukhammad – Praised
52. Murad – Desire
53. Musa – Saved from the water
54. Nasriddin – Victory of religion
55. Navruz – New day
56. Nazir – Observer
57. Nemat – Blessing
58. Nodir – Rare
59. Nuriddin – Light of religion
60. Olim – Scholar
61. Orzubek – Heart's desire
62. Parviz – Victorious
63. Qahramon – Hero
64. Qobil – Able
65. Rahim – Merciful
66. Rajab – Seventh month of the Islamic calendar
67. Rasul – Messenger
68. Rustam – Strong, brave
69. Sabir – Patient

70. Said – Happy
71. Sardor – Leader
72. Shamsiddin – Sun of religion
73. Sherzod – Lion's son
74. Shohruh – Famous
75. Shuhrat – Fame
76. Sirojiddin – Light of religion
77. Sobir – Patient
78. Suhrob – Water of life
79. Sulaymon – Man of peace
80. Tolib – Seeker
81. Tohir – Pure
82. Umar – Life
83. Umid – Hope
84. Utkir – Bright
85. Vahid – Unique
86. Valijon – Power of youth
87. Vohid – Unique
88. Xurshid – Sun
89. Yaqub – Supplanter
90. Yorqin – Bright
91. Yusuf – God will add
92. Zafar – Victory
93. Ziyovuddin – Beauty of religion
94. Zokir – Remembrance
95. Sherali – Lion king
96. Shodmon – Happy heart
97. Nasim – Breeze
98. Roshan – Bright, light
99. Qudrat – Power, strength
100. Rahmat – Mercy

Kyrgyzstani baby boy names

1. Adilet – Justice
2. Akylbek – Wise ruler
3. Almaz – Diamond
4. Amanbek – Peaceful ruler
5. Arslan – Lion
6. Asanali – Easy-going
7. Askar – Soldier
8. Azamat – Greatness
9. Aziz – Powerful
10. Baktiyar – Fortunate
11. Batyr – Brave
12. Bekbolot – Generous
13. Bekzat – Desire to be supreme
14. Bolot – Steel
15. Cholpon – Venus or morning star
16. Daniyar – Wise and strong
17. Dastan – Story
18. Doolot – Wealth
19. Edil – Noble
20. Eldiyar – Independent
21. Emir – Prince
22. Erkin – Free
23. Ermek – Wish, desire
24. Ernazar – Generous
25. Farkhad – Happy
26. Faruh – Happy, joyous
27. Galib – Winner
28. Gulzar – Rose garden
29. Ibragim – Father of many
30. Ilias – The Lord is my God
31. Iskander – Defender of mankind
32. Jantoro – Life force
33. Jusup – He will add

34. Kanat – Wing
35. Kanybek – Master of the soul
36. Kasym – Divided
37. Kudaybergen – Given by God
38. Kurmanbek – Steady ruler
39. Madamin – My diamond
40. Marat – Wish, desire
41. Mars – God of War
42. Meder – Friend
43. Meerim – Kindness
44. Murat – Wish, desire
45. Nurbek – Light ruler
46. Oktom – Eight
47. Omurbek – Long-lived ruler
48. Orozbek – Mountain ruler
49. Osmon – Heaven
50. Raimbek – Rich ruler
51. Rasul – Messenger
52. Rustam – Brave, bold
53. Sagyn – Praise
54. Sanjar – Prince, king
55. Saparbek – Pure ruler
56. Sardarbek – Leader ruler
57. Shamil – Comprehensive, universal
58. Sultan – Ruler, king
59. Tair – Bird
60. Talant – Talent
61. Talgat – Full moon
62. Talip – Seeker, student
63. Tamerlan – Iron ruler
64. Tash – Stone
65. Tynchtykbek – Happy ruler
66. Ulan – Warrior
67. Umar – Long-lived
68. Urmat – Wish, desire
69. Usen – Brave

70. Uulu – Son of
71. Vali – Governor
72. Yrysbek – Light ruler
73. Zafar – Victory
74. Zaman – Time, age
75. Zhanibek – Soul ruler
76. Zhanybek – New ruler
77. Zhasur – Brave
78. Zhenish – Owner, master
79. Zholaman – Free man
80. Zhunus – Generous
81. Ziyat – Growth, increase
82. Abay – Carefree
83. Adil – Just, fair
84. Aibek – Moon ruler
85. Akjol – White light
86. Altynbek – Golden ruler
87. Aman – Peace
88. Anarbek – Pomegranate ruler
89. Aziret – Noble
90. Baatyr – Hero, brave
91. Baglan – Tiger
92. Baktiar – Lucky, fortunate
93. Batu – Loyal, firm
94. Bolotbek – Steel ruler
95. Chingiz – World ruler
96. Dastanbek – Story ruler
97. Eldos – Independent
98. Emil – Industrious, striving
99. Ernist – Serious
100. Fazil – Excellent, generous

Turkmenistani baby boy names

1. Abadan - Eternal
2. Abay - Calm
3. Ada - Island
4. Adal - Noble
5. Agajan - Noble Soul
6. Akja - White Soul
7. Altyn - Gold
8. Annaguly - Noble Rose
9. Arslan - Lion
10. Aşgabat - Love City
11. Aşk - Love
12. Ata - Father
13. Azat - Free
14. Baýram - Festival
15. Begli - Prince
16. Berdi - Strong
17. Berdimyrat - Strong Belief
18. Çary - Wizard
19. Däneş - Knowledge
20. Döwlet - State
21. Edebi - Literary
22. Enejan - Soul Mother
23. Ertir - Brave
24. Esen - Healthy
25. Farhad - Happiness
26. Gahryman - Hero
27. Gara - Black
28. Garaja - Black Soul
29. Gurbanguly - Blessed by God
30. Gurbanmyrat - Blessed Belief
31. Gül - Rose
32. Hally - Lucky
33. Hemra - Joy

34. Hoja - Teacher
35. Hydyr - Green
36. Ilham - Inspiration
37. Ilyas - The Lord is my God
38. Inanç - Faith
39. Ismail - God will hear
40. Jahan - World
41. Jemal - Beauty
42. Kanat - Wing
43. Kerim - Generous
44. Kömek - Help
45. Mahtumkuli - Blessed Poet
46. Marat - Desire
47. Merdan - Man
48. Meylis - Gathering
49. Muhamed - Praised
50. Murad - Desire
51. Myrat - Desire
52. Niyaz - Need
53. Nurmuhammet - Light of Mohammed
54. Ogul - Son
55. Oraz - Fortune
56. Orazgeldi - Fortune has come
57. Paygambar - Prophet
58. Pir - Old
59. Rahim - Merciful
60. Rahmet - Mercy
61. Rejep - Respect
62. Rovşen - Light
63. Sähet - Health
64. Sapar - Journey
65. Serdar - Leader
66. Seyit - Prince
67. Şamyrat - Famous Belief
68. Şatlyk - Happiness
69. Şir - Lion

70. Sohbet - Conversation
71. Söýgi - Love
72. Süleýman - Peace
73. Tagan - Blacksmith
74. Täjigul - Crown Rose
75. Togrul - Falcon
76. Toý - Feast
77. Türkmen - Turkmen
78. Umid - Hope
79. Watan - Homeland
80. Weli - Saint
81. Wepa - Glory
82. Yalkap - Companion
83. Yigit - Brave
84. Yslam - Islam
85. Ysmammet - Heard by Mohammed
86. Zohre - Venus
87. Zülfikar - Cleaver of the Spine
88. Aman - Peace
89. Batyr - Hero
90. Bayram - Festival
91. Chary - Wizard
92. Dovlet - State
93. Ertir - Brave
94. Gahryman - Hero
95. Gara - Black
96. Garaja - Black soul
97. Hally - Lucky
98. Hemra - Joy
99. Kanat - Wing
100. Kerim - Generous

Mongolian baby boy names

1. Altan - Gold
2. Batbayar - Strong Joy
3. Tömörbaatar - Iron Hero
4. Chuluunbold - Stone Steel
5. Erdene - Jewel
6. Ganbaatar - Steel Hero
7. Khosbayar - Happy River
8. Mönkhbat - Eternal Firmness
9. Naranbaatar - Sun Hero
10. Otgonbayar - Youngest Joy
11. Sükhbaatar - Axe Hero
12. Tsend-Ayush - Long Health
13. Ulziibayar - Buddha's Joy
14. Zorig - Brave
15. Agvaan - Holy
16. Bat-Erdene - Strong Jewel
17. Chuluun - Stone
18. Delger - Wide, Expansive
19. Enkhjargal - Peace Blessing
20. Gantulga - Steel Hearth
21. Khulan - Onager
22. Munkh-Orgil - Eternal Brave
23. Narantsetseg - Sun Flower
24. Oyuunchimeg - Wisdom Ornament
25. Sükh-Ochir - Axe Victory
26. Tserendorj - Strength of the Buddha
27. Ulzii - Luck
28. Zorigtbaatar - Brave Hero
29. Amgalan - Peace, Calm
30. Batjargal - Strong Happiness
31. Chuluunbaatar - Stone Hero
32. Delgermurun - Wide River
33. Enkhtaivan - Peaceful

34. Ganbold - Steel Firm
35. Khurelbaatar - Wheel Hero
36. Munkhtur - Eternal Buddha
37. Naran - Sun
38. Oyun - Intellect
39. Sükhbat - Axe Firm
40. Tseren - Buddha
41. Unen - Truth
42. Zul - Iron
43. Anand - Happiness
44. Batkhuyag - Strong Blessing
45. Dagvadorj - Steel Buddha
46. Delgertsetseg - Wide Flower
47. Enkhbold - Peaceful Firm
48. Ganzorig - Steel Brave
49. Khurts - Steel
50. Munkh-Erdene - Eternal Jewel
51. Naranbaatar - Sun Hero
52. Oyunchimeg - Wisdom Ornament
53. Sükhgerel - Axe Light
54. Tserendash - Strength Stone
55. Uuganbayar - Youngest Joy
56. Zulaa - Iron
57. Ankhbayar - Blessing Joy
58. Batmönkh - Strong Eternal
59. Davaajargal - Happiness
60. Delgerjargal - Wide Happiness
61. Enkhjargal - Peace Blessing
62. Gantumur - Steel Iron
63. Khurel - Wheel
64. Munkhjargal - Eternal Blessing
65. Narangerel - Sun Light
66. Oyuun - Wisdom
67. Sükhmönkh - Axe Eternal
68. Tserendorj - Strength Buddha
69. Uurtsaikh - Youngest River

70. Zulbat - Iron Firm
71. Ankhtsetseg - Blessing Flower
72. Batnasan - Strong Buddha
73. Davaasuren - Happiness Long Life
74. Delgertogtokh - Wide Steel
75. Enkhmaa - Peace Mother
76. Ganzul - Steel Iron
77. Khurelee - Wheel
78. Munkhochir - Eternal Victory
79. Narantuya - Sun Ray
80. Oyuunerdene - Wisdom Jewel
81. Sükhochir - Axe Victory
82. Tserenbat - Buddha Firm
83. Uuganaa - Youngest
84. Zuljargal - Iron Happiness
85. Ankhtuya - Blessing Ray
86. Bat-Ochir - Strong Victory
87. Davaasuren - Happiness Long Life
88. Delgersaikhan - Wide Good
89. Enkhzul - Peace Iron
90. Gantugs - Steel
91. Khurelbaatar - Wheel Hero
92. Munkhtsetseg - Eternal Flower
93. Narantungalag - Sun Light
94. Oyuungerel - Wisdom Light
95. Sükhochir - Axe Victory
96. Tserenchimed - Buddha Ornament
97. Uuganbaatar - Youngest Hero
98. Zulzaya - Iron Fate
99. Ankhtur - Blessing Buddha
100. Bat-Orgil - Strong Brave

Vietnamese baby boy names

1. An - Peace
2. Bao - Protection
3. Cadeo - Folk song
4. Dang - Dignity
5. Dat - Accomplished
6. Duc - Moral, good
7. Giang - River
8. Hai - Two or second
9. Hien - Gentle, nice
10. Huy - Glory
11. Khoa - Science or knowledge
12. Khai - Beginning or open
13. Khanh - Success
14. Lam - Forest
15. Luan - Ethics
16. Minh - Bright
17. Nam - South
18. Nghia - Righteousness
19. Phong - Wind
20. Quang - Clear, bright
21. Sang - Noble
22. Tan - New
23. Thanh - Clear, bright
24. Trung - Loyal
25. Tuan - Intelligent
26. Vinh - Glory
27. Vu - Rain
28. Xuan - Spring
29. Yen - Peaceful
30. Anh - Bright
31. Binh - Peaceful
32. Chien - Battle
33. Dinh - Summit

34. Duong - Virile
35. Hao - Good
36. Hung - Heroic
37. Kien - Strong
38. Lanh - Cold
39. Nhan - Kind
40. Phuc - Happiness
41. Quyen - Power
42. Son - Mountain
43. Thien - Heaven
44. Toan - Whole
45. Vien - Complete
46. Thang - Victory
47. Tri - Intelligence
48. Tung - Pine tree
49. Vuong - King
50. Hoang - Royal
51. Huy - Bright
52. Kiet - Honor
53. Long - Dragon
54. Mau - Fast
55. Nhat - Sun
56. Phu - Wealthy
57. Quoc - Nation
58. Thao - Respectful
59. Tien - Fairy
60. Van - Literature
61. Thanh - Bright
62. Hoa - Flower
63. Dien - Genius
64. Giau - Rich
65. Hieu - Understanding
66. Khang - Health
67. Loc - Blessing
68. Ninh - Peaceful
69. Phuong - Direction

70. Quy - Precious
71. Thuan - Agree
72. Truong - Long-lasting
73. Vui - Joyful
74. Hau - Generous
75. Khoa - Knowledge
76. Luan - Discussion
77. Minh - Bright
78. Ngoc - Gem
79. Phan - Glory
80. Quan - Army
81. Thong - Smart
82. Truc - Bamboo
83. Vinh - Glory
84. Hoc - Learning
85. Kiet - Honor
86. Lap - Independent
87. Manh - Strong
88. Nguyet - Moon
89. Phuc - Blessing
90. Quy - Precious
91. Tho - Longevity
92. Trung - Loyal
93. Vi - Precious
94. Hien - Gentle
95. Kien - Build
96. Linh - Spirit
97. Mau - Fast
98. Nghia - Righteousness
99. Phuoc - Blessed
100. Quang - Light

Thai baby boy names

1. Adisorn - 'extraordinary or superior'
2. Akara - 'the letter'
3. Amorn - 'love'
4. Anan - 'cloud'
5. Anuchit - 'the chosen one'
6. Anuman - 'small, diminutive'
7. Arthit - 'sun'
8. Atid - 'sun'
9. Boon-Mee - 'lucky'
10. Boon-Nam - 'born with good fortune'
11. Chai - 'victory'
12. Chaiya - 'triumph'
13. Chakri - 'emperor'
14. Chalerm - 'celebrated'
15. Chanchai - 'victory'
16. Channarong - 'experienced warrior'
17. Charan - 'life'
18. Chatri - 'brave knight'
19. Chavalit - 'excellent knight'
20. Chayan - 'intelligent'
21. Chul - 'something that is loved'
22. Darunee - 'good view'
23. Decha - 'power'
24. Ekachai - 'victorious'
25. Ekamai - 'intelligent'
26. Fai - 'fire'
27. Ganya - 'knowledgeable'
28. Harit - 'green'
29. Inthira - 'a very wealthy person'
30. Isra - 'freedom'
31. Itthi - 'powerful'
32. Jirayu - 'excellent splendor'
33. Kanda - 'beloved'

34. Kasem - 'happiness'
35. Kiet - 'honor'
36. Kittisak - 'honorable friend'
37. Kongdej - 'powerful'
38. Kraisorn - 'pride'
39. Krung - 'city'
40. Lamon - 'gentle'
41. Manop - 'magnificent'
42. Manuch - 'man'
43. Mayuree - 'emerald'
44. Mee Noi - 'little bear'
45. Niran - 'eternal'
46. Noppadol - 'noble'
47. Pairoj - 'jewel'
48. Pan - 'a thousand'
49. Panupong - 'thousand of success'
50. Panya - 'knowledge'
51. Pichai - 'noble'
52. Pramuan - 'approval'
53. Prasert - 'excellent'
54. Pravit - 'honorable'
55. Preecha - 'intelligence'
56. Pridi - 'joyful'
57. Putt - 'Buddha'
58. Rangsey - 'seven colors'
59. Ratan - 'jewel'
60. Ritthirong - 'righteous warrior'
61. Ruam - 'together'
62. Sakda - 'power'
63. Samart - 'capable'
64. San - 'peaceful'
65. Sanya - 'worthy of honor'
66. Sarit - 'diamond'
67. Sermchai - 'victory'
68. Settawut - 'worthy of love'
69. Siwakorn - 'good destiny'

70. Somchai - 'man of worth'
71. Somwang - 'hope'
72. Songkran - 'passage of the sun'
73. Sritong - 'golden glory'
74. Suksan - 'happiness'
75. Sumalee - 'beautiful flower'
76. Sunan - 'good word'
77. Surin - 'good deed'
78. Tan - 'new'
79. Tanawat - 'endless area'
80. Thaksin - 'south'
81. Than - 'million'
82. Thanakorn - 'record of a million'
83. Thawat - 'tradition'
84. Thongchai - 'golden victory'
85. Thongkhao - 'white gold'
86. Thonglek - 'small gold'
87. Thunwa - 'dawn'
88. Ti - 'wealth'
89. Tida - 'daughter'
90. Tong - 'gold'
91. Trong - 'strength'
92. Udom - 'the best'
93. Veera - 'brave'
94. Virote - 'great'
95. Viroj - 'excellent'
96. Wann - 'desire'
97. Wannarat - 'desired jewel'
98. Wissanu - 'knowledgeable'
99. Wit - 'intelligent'
100. Yod - 'excellent'

Malaysian baby boy names

1. Aariz – Leader, ruler
2. Adli – Just, fair
3. Afiq – Honest, upright
4. Aiman – Blessed, lucky
5. Akmal – Perfect, complete
6. Alif – Friendly, sociable
7. Amir – Prince, commander
8. Arif – Knowledgeable, wise
9. Asyraf – Noble, respected
10. Azim – Determined, resolved
11. Badrul – Full moon
12. Basir – Insightful, perceptive
13. Danish – Knowledge, wisdom
14. Dzul – Possessor, master
15. Ehsan – Charitable, compassionate
16. Faiz – Victorious, successful
17. Firdaus – Paradise, heaven
18. Ghazi – Warrior, conqueror
19. Hafiz – Protector, guardian
20. Haris – Vigilant, watchful
21. Idris – Studious, learned
22. Ikram – Honor, hospitality
23. Imran – Prosperity, happiness
24. Irfan – Gratitude, thankfulness
25. Iskandar – Defender of mankind
26. Jamal – Beauty, grace
27. Kamal – Perfection, excellence
28. Karim – Generous, noble
29. Latif – Gentle, kind
30. Lukman – Wise, learned
31. Mahir – Skilled, proficient
32. Malik – King, sovereign
33. Mansur – Victorious, triumphant

34. Naufal – Generous, noble
35. Nizam – Order, arrangement
36. Qasim – Distributor, divider
37. Rafiq – Gentle, kind
38. Rauf – Merciful, compassionate
39. Saif – Sword, saber
40. Salman – Safe, secure
41. Tariq – Morning star
42. Ubaid – Faithful, devoted
43. Wafi – Faithful, loyal
44. Yasin – A chapter of the Quran
45. Zahir – Bright, shining
46. Zaki – Pure, chaste
47. Zulfikar – The sword of Ali
48. Aqil – Intelligent, wise
49. Basyar – Bringer of glad tidings
50. Daud – Beloved, dear
51. Farid – Unique, singular
52. Ghaffar – Forgiving, merciful
53. Hamid – Praiseworthy, commendable
54. Ikhwan – Brotherhood, fraternity
55. Jalil – Great, revered
56. Kadir – Powerful, capable
57. Latif – Gentle, kind
58. Majid – Glorious, noble
59. Nasir – Helper, supporter
60. Omar – Life, long living
61. Qadir – Capable, powerful
62. Rais – Captain, chief
63. Samir – Companion, entertainer
64. Tahir – Pure, clean
65. Umar – Life, long living
66. Wazir – Minister, counselor
67. Yasir – Wealthy, prosperous
68. Zafar – Victory, triumph
69. Zuhair – Bright, shining

70. Fahim – Understanding, intelligent
71. Hakim – Wise, judicious
72. Ihsan – Beneficence, charity
73. Jalal – Majesty, grandeur
74. Kamran – Successful, prosperous
75. Lutfi – Kind, gentle
76. Mubarak – Blessed, fortunate
77. Naim – Comfort, tranquility
78. Qayyum – Self-sustaining, eternal
79. Rashid – Rightly guided, mature
80. Suhail – Easy, uncomplicated
81. Taufik – Success, prosperity
82. Uthman – Companion of Prophet Muhammad
83. Wahid – Unique, singular
84. Yaqub – Supplanter, successor
85. Zain – Beauty, grace
86. Faisal – Judge, arbitrator
87. Hakimi – Wise, judicious
88. Izhar – Expression, manifestation
89. Jalil – Great, revered
90. Khairul – The best of
91. Luqman – Wise, learned
92. Muhsin – Beneficent, charitable
93. Nabil – Noble, generous
94. Qamar – Moon, satellite
95. Ridwan – Pleasure, satisfaction
96. Syafiq – Compassionate, tender
97. Talib – Seeker, student
98. Usman – Baby bustard
99. Wajdi – Passionate, ardent
100. Yazid – Increasing, growing

Indonesian baby boy names

1. Aditya – The sun
2. Agus – Good
3. Ahmad – Highly praised
4. Akbar – Great
5. Ali – Exalted
6. Andi – Warrior
7. Andika – Large; Great
8. Angga – Handsome
9. Anwar – Luminous
10. Arief – Wise
11. Arjuna – Bright; shining
12. Arya – Noble
13. Bagas – Strong
14. Bambang – Knight
15. Bayu – Wind
16. Beni – Blessed
17. Bima – Brave
18. Bram – God's gift
19. Budi – Reason; mind
20. Cahya – Light
21. Damar – Light
22. Dani – God is my judge
23. Darma – Duty; law
24. Dedi – Beloved
25. Dika – One who is strong
26. Dimas – Sunset
27. Doni – World ruler
28. Dwi – Second; twin
29. Edi – Wealthy
30. Eko – First child
31. Fajar – Dawn
32. Fikri – Thought; intellect
33. Galang – To prepare

34. Gilang – Shining
35. Hadi – Guide to righteousness
36. Hamid – Praiseworthy
37. Hanif – True believer
38. Haris – Guardian
39. Hasan – Handsome
40. Hendra – King of kings
41. Iman – Faith
42. Indra – God of rain and thunder
43. Irfan – Gratitude
44. Iskandar – Defender of mankind
45. Jaka – Young man
46. Jamal – Beauty
47. Joko – Elder brother
48. Kadek – Little brother
49. Kamil – Perfect
50. Kusuma – Flower
51. Lintang – Star
52. Lukman – Wise
53. Mahesa – Great
54. Malik – King
55. Mulya – Valuable
56. Nanda – Joy
57. Nizar – Rare
58. Nusa – Island
59. Pasha – Pass
60. Putra – Son
61. Raden – Title for Javanese nobility
62. Rahmad – Merciful
63. Raka – Full moon
64. Rama – Pleasing
65. Reza – Contentment
66. Rizki – Blessing
67. Sakti – Power
68. Salman – Safe
69. Samudra – Ocean

70. Sandi – Defender
71. Satria – Knight
72. Surya – Sun
73. Tama – Perfect
74. Tegar – Firm
75. Tirta – Holy water
76. Umar – Life
77. Utama – Main
78. Wibowo – Handsome
79. Wira – Hero
80. Wisnu – Preserver
81. Yuda – War
82. Yudha – Warrior
83. Yuli – Youthful
84. Yuni – Handsome
85. Zain – Good; beautiful
86. Zaki – Pure
87. Zidan – Growth
88. Abyan – Clear; eloquent
89. Adil – Fair; just
90. Ahsan – Most beautiful
91. Akmal – Perfect
92. Alif – Friendly; sociable
93. Aman – Safe; secure
94. Amin – Faithful; trustworthy
95. Amir – Prince; leader
96. Arif – Wise; intelligent
97. Asif – Gather; harvest
98. Asim – Protector; guardian
99. Aziz – Mighty; powerful
100. Badar – Full moon

Filipino baby boy names

1. Adonis – Lord
2. Adrian – Dark
3. Agapito – Beloved
4. Agustin – Majestic
5. Alberto – Noble
6. Alejandro – Defender
7. Alfonso – Noble and ready
8. Alfredo – Wise counselor
9. Alon – Wave
10. Alvaro – Guardian
11. Amado – Loved
12. Amihan – Northeast wind
13. Andres – Manly
14. Antonio – Priceless
15. Apolinario – Follower of Apollo
16. Armando – Soldier
17. Arturo – Bear
18. Bayani – Hero
19. Benigno – Kind
20. Benjamin – Son of the right hand
21. Bernardo – Brave bear
22. Carlos – Free man
23. Cesar – Hairy
24. Danilo – God is my judge
25. Dante – Enduring
26. Dario – Wealthy
27. David – Beloved
28. Diego – Supplanter
29. Dionisio – God of wine
30. Eduardo – Wealthy guardian
31. Emilio – Rival
32. Enrique – Home ruler
33. Ernesto – Serious

34. Eugenio – Well-born
35. Felipe – Lover of horses
36. Fernando – Adventurous
37. Francisco – Free man
38. Gabriel – God is my strength
39. Galo – Rooster
40. Gregorio – Watchful
41. Guillermo – Will helmet
42. Hector – Holding fast
43. Ignacio – Fiery
44. Isagani – Fruitful
45. Jaime – Supplanter
46. Javier – Bright
47. Jericho – City of the moon
48. Jesus – God is salvation
49. Joaquin – God will establish
50. Jose – He will add
51. Juan – God is gracious
52. Julio – Youthful
53. Kiko – Free man
54. Lando – Famous throughout the land
55. Lito – Joyful
56. Lorenzo – From Laurentum
57. Lucas – From Lucania
58. Luis – Famous warrior
59. Magtanggol – To defend
60. Manuel – God is with us
61. Marco – Warlike
62. Mario – Male
63. Mateo – Gift of God
64. Miguel – Who is like God?
65. Nardo – Strong
66. Narciso – Sleep
67. Nestor – Homecoming
68. Nicolo – Victory of the people
69. Orlando – Famous throughout the land

70. Oscar – Friend of deer
71. Pablo – Small
72. Paco – Free man
73. Pancho – Free man
74. Paolo – Small
75. Patricio – Nobleman
76. Pedro – Rock
77. Rafael – God has healed
78. Ramon – Wise protector
79. Ricardo – Powerful ruler
80. Roberto – Bright fame
81. Rodrigo – Famous ruler
82. Rolando – Famous throughout the land
83. Romulo – Citizen of Rome
84. Rosario – Rosary
85. Ruben – Behold, a son
86. Salvador – Savior
87. Sancho – Holy
88. Santiago – Supplanter
89. Santos – Saints
90. Sergio – Servant
91. Simplicio – Simple
92. Teodoro – Gift of God
93. Tito – Giant
94. Tomas – Twin
95. Vicente – Conquering
96. Victor – Conqueror
97. Vincente – Conquering
98. Waldo – Rule
99. Xander – Defender of the people
100. Zacarias – God has remembered

Singaporean baby boy names

1. Aiden – Fiery
2. Brandon – From the broom hill
3. Caleb – Faithful, bold
4. Dylan – Son of the sea
5. Ethan – Strong, firm
6. Firdaus – Paradise
7. Gabriel – God is my strength
8. Haikal – Story, tale
9. Irfan – Knowledge, learning
10. Jasper – Treasurer
11. Kai – Ocean
12. Liam – Strong-willed warrior
13. Matthew – Gift of God
14. Noah – Rest, peace
15. Oliver – Olive tree
16. Preston – Priest's town
17. Qadir – Capable, powerful
18. Ryan – Little king
19. Samuel – God has heard
20. Tristan – Tumult
21. Umar – Life, long living
22. Vincent – Conqueror
23. Wyatt – Brave in war
24. Xavier – New house
25. Yusuf – God will add
26. Zachary – The Lord has remembered
27. Aaron – High mountain
28. Benjamin – Son of the right hand
29. Charles – Free man
30. Daniel – God is my judge
31. Edwin – Rich friend
32. Farhan – Happy, joyous
33. George – Farmer

34. Harry – Army ruler
35. Isaac – He will laugh
36. Justin – Just, fair
37. Kelvin – River man
38. Lucas – Light
39. Marcus – Warlike
40. Nathan – He gave
41. Oscar – Friend of deer
42. Patrick – Nobleman
43. Quentin – Fifth
44. Russell – Redhead
45. Stephen – Crown
46. Timothy – Honoring God
47. Uzair – Helper, strength
48. Victor – Winner
49. William – Resolute protector
50. Xavier – Bright, splendid
51. Yohannes – God is gracious
52. Zain – Beauty, grace
53. Adam – Man, to make
54. Brian – High, noble
55. Colin – Young creature
56. Derek – The people's ruler
57. Eric – Eternal ruler
58. Felix – Happy, fortunate
59. Gavin – White hawk
60. Howard – High guardian
61. Ivan – God is gracious
62. Jack – God is gracious
63. Kenneth – Handsome
64. Leonard – Brave lion
65. Michael – Who is like God?
66. Norman – Northman
67. Owen – Young warrior
68. Paul – Small
69. Quincy – Estate of the fifth son

70. Roger – Famous spear
71. Simon – The listener
72. Thomas – Twin
73. Upton – High town
74. Vernon – Springlike
75. Walter – Army ruler
76. Xavier – Bright, splendid
77. Yosef – God will increase
78. Zephyr – West wind
79. Andrew – Manly, brave
80. Bruce – From the brushwood thicket
81. Clifford – Ford by a cliff
82. David – Beloved
83. Edward – Wealthy guardian
84. Francis – Frenchman
85. Gerald – Ruler with the spear
86. Harold – Army power
87. Ian – God is gracious
88. James – Supplanter
89. Kevin – Gentle, kind
90. Lawrence – From Laurentum
91. Martin – Warlike
92. Nigel – Champion
93. Orson – Bear cub
94. Peter – Stone
95. Quentin – Fifth
96. Richard – Brave ruler
97. Stanley – Stone clearing
98. Terence – Tender, gracious
99. Ulysses – Wrathful
100. Vincent – Conquering

Laotian baby boy names

1. Aiden – 'little fire'
2. Boun – 'merit'
3. Chai – 'alive'
4. Daeng – 'red'
5. Ekalavya – 'student of Drona'
6. Fai – 'fire'
7. Gai – 'chicken'
8. Hai – 'sea'
9. Ithan – 'enduring, long-lived'
10. Jai – 'victory'
11. Kham – 'gold'
12. Lai – 'lion'
13. Mani – 'gem'
14. Nai – 'serpent'
15. Oudom – 'superior'
16. Pao – 'duck'
17. Quan – 'spring of water'
18. Rith – 'truth'
19. Somsak – 'born on Saturday'
20. Tan – 'new'
21. Un – 'intelligent'
22. Vai – 'water'
23. Wai – 'water'
24. Xay – 'victory'
25. Yai – 'big'
26. Zai – 'victory'
27. Ake – 'ancestor'
28. Bounthanh – 'meritorious progress'
29. Chantho – 'famous'
30. Daeng – 'red'
31. Ekkarat – 'democratic'
32. Fai – 'fire'
33. Gai – 'chicken'

34. Hai – 'ocean'
35. Ithan – 'enduring'
36. Jai – 'victory'
37. Kham – 'gold'
38. Lai – 'lion'
39. Mani – 'gem'
40. Nai – 'serpent'
41. Oudom – 'superior'
42. Pao – 'duck'
43. Quan – 'spring of water'
44. Rith – 'truth'
45. Somsak – 'born on Saturday'
46. Tan – 'new'
47. Un – 'intelligent'
48. Vai – 'water'
49. Wai – 'water'
50. Xay – 'victory'
51. Yai – 'big'
52. Zai – 'victory'
53. Ake – 'ancestor'
54. Bounthanh – 'meritorious progress'
55. Chantho – 'famous'
56. Daeng – 'red'
57. Ekkarat – 'democratic'
58. Fai – 'fire'
59. Gai – 'chicken'
60. Hai – 'ocean'
61. Ithan – 'enduring'
62. Jai – 'victory'
63. Kham – 'gold'
64. Lai – 'lion'
65. Mani – 'gem'
66. Nai – 'serpent'
67. Oudom – 'superior'
68. Pao – 'duck'
69. Quan – 'spring of water'

70. Rith – 'truth'
71. Somsak – 'born on Saturday'
72. Tan – 'new'
73. Un – 'intelligent'
74. Vai – 'water'
75. Wai – 'water'
76. Xay – 'victory'
77. Yai – 'big'
78. Zai – 'victory'
79. Ake – 'ancestor'
80. Bounthanh – 'meritorious progress'
81. Chantho – 'famous'
82. Daeng – 'red'
83. Ekkarat – 'democratic'
84. Fai – 'fire'
85. Gai – 'chicken'
86. Hai – 'ocean'
87. Ithan – 'enduring'
88. Jai – 'victory'
89. Kham – 'gold'
90. Lai – 'lion'
91. Mani – 'gem'
92. Nai – 'serpent'
93. Oudom – 'superior'
94. Pao – 'duck'
95. Quan – 'spring of water'
96. Rith – 'truth'
97. Somsak – 'born on Saturday'
98. Tan – 'new'
99. Un – 'intelligent'
100. Vai – 'water'

Bruneian baby boy names

1. Aiman – 'blessed' or 'fortunate'
2. Akif – 'devoted' or 'dedicated'
3. Alif – 'friendly' and 'sociable'
4. Ammar – 'virtuous', 'devout' or 'long-lived'
5. Azim – 'determined' or 'resolute'
6. Bahri – 'of the sea'
7. Basir – 'wise' or 'sagacious'
8. Daud – 'beloved'
9. Fadil – 'generous' or 'honorable'
10. Ghazi – 'warrior' or 'champion'
11. Hadi – 'leader' or 'guide'
12. Idris – 'interpreter'
13. Jafar – 'stream' or 'river'
14. Kamal – 'perfection'
15. Latif – 'kind' or 'gentle'
16. Malik – 'king' or 'sovereign'
17. Nasir – 'helper' or 'supporter'
18. Omar – 'life' or 'long-lived'
19. Qasim – 'one who distributes'
20. Rafiq – 'friend' or 'companion'
21. Saad – 'happiness' or 'good fortune'
22. Tahir – 'pure' or 'chaste'
23. Ubaid – 'small slave'
24. Wafi – 'faithful' or 'loyal'
25. Yasin – Name of a chapter in the Quran
26. Zahir – 'bright' or 'shining'
27. Adil – 'just' or 'fair'
28. Badr – 'full moon'
29. Faisal – 'decisive' or 'judge'
30. Hakim – 'wise' or 'ruler'
31. Irfan – 'knowledge' or 'awareness'
32. Jalil – 'great' or 'revered'
33. Kamil – 'perfect' or 'complete'

34. Luqman – 'wise'
35. Majid – 'glorious' or 'noble'
36. Nabil – 'noble' or 'generous'
37. Qadir – 'capable' or 'powerful'
38. Rashid – 'rightly guided' or 'having true faith'
39. Samir – 'entertaining companion'
40. Tariq – 'morning star'
41. Umar – 'flourishing' or 'thriving'
42. Wahid – 'unique' or 'singular'
43. Yasir – 'wealthy' or 'successful'
44. Zahid – 'ascetic' or 'devout'
45. Adnan – 'settler'
46. Bilal – 'water' or 'moisture'
47. Faris – 'horseman' or 'knight'
48. Hamza – 'strong' or 'steadfast'
49. Imran – 'prosperity' or 'happiness'
50. Jamal – 'beauty'
51. Khalid – 'eternal' or 'immortal'
52. Mansur – 'victorious' or 'triumphant'
53. Naim – 'blessing' or 'favour'
54. Qais – 'firm' or 'hard'
55. Rauf – 'compassionate' or 'merciful'
56. Sufyan – 'fast-moving' or 'light-footed'
57. Talib – 'seeker' or 'student'
58. Usman – 'baby bustard' (a type of bird)
59. Wajid – 'finder' or 'inventor'
60. Yaqub – 'supplanter'
61. Zain – 'beauty' or 'grace'
62. Aqil – 'intelligent' or 'wise'
63. Bari – 'creator'
64. Fahim – 'understanding' or 'intelligent'
65. Haris – 'guardian' or 'protector'
66. Izzat – 'honour' or 'glory'
67. Jazib – 'beautiful' or 'handsome'
68. Khair – 'good' or 'blessing'
69. Marwan – 'solid' or 'flint'

70. Naufal – 'generous' or 'bountiful'
71. Qamar – 'moon'
72. Rais – 'captain' or 'chief'
73. Sajid – 'one who prostrates'
74. Taufiq – 'success' or 'prosperity'
75. Uzair – 'helper' or 'supporter'
76. Wajih – 'distinguished' or 'eminent'
77. Yamin – 'right' or 'true'
78. Ziyad – 'growth' or 'progress'
79. Asif – 'gather' or 'harvest'
80. Baha – 'splendour' or 'glory'
81. Fakhr – 'pride' or 'glory'
82. Hasan – 'handsome' or 'good'
83. Iqbal – 'prosperity' or 'success'
84. Jalal – 'majesty' or 'glory'
85. Karim – 'generous' or 'noble'
86. Mahir – 'skilled' or 'expert'
87. Nizar – 'rare' or 'precious'
88. Qudrat – 'power' or 'might'
89. Rahim – 'merciful' or 'compassionate'
90. Salim – 'safe' or 'sound'
91. Tawfiq – 'success' or 'reconciliation'
92. Uthman – 'baby snake'
93. Waleed – 'newborn'
94. Yusra – 'prosperity' or 'wealth'
95. Zulfiqar – The name of the sword of Ali in the Islamic tradition
96. Ashraf – 'most noble' or 'honourable'
97. Burhan – 'proof' or 'evidence'
98. Faiz – 'victor' or 'successful'
99. Hafiz – 'guardian' or 'memorizer'
100. Iskandar – The Arabic form of Alexander, 'defender of mankind'

Taiwanese baby boy names

1. Aiden – little fire
2. Bao – treasure
3. Cai – wealth
4. Duan – section, piece
5. Enlai – favor coming
6. Fai – beginning
7. Genghis – right, just
8. Hao – good, perfect
9. Imin – intelligence
10. Jia – good, fine
11. Kai – victory
12. Li – strong
13. Min – quick
14. Nianzu – thinking of ancestors
15. Ong – peace
16. Ping – stable
17. Qiang – strong
18. Rong – glory
19. Shen – deep thinker
20. Tai – great
21. Ushi – ox
22. Vui – joyful
23. Wei – power
24. Xing – star
25. Yong – brave
26. Zhi – ambitious
27. Aiguo – patriotic
28. Bo – precious
29. Chao – surpassing
30. De – virtue
31. Fung – wind
32. Guozhi – may the state govern
33. Huan – happy, joyous

34. Jian – healthy
35. Kang – healthy
36. Lei – thunder
37. Ming – bright
38. Niu – ox
39. Peng – rock
40. Qiu – autumn
41. Ru – scholar
42. Shui – water
43. Tian – field
44. Uen – culture, writing
45. Wei – big, great
46. Xiu – elegant
47. Yao – bright, shining
48. Zhen – precious
49. An – peace
50. Bing – soldier
51. Chen – great
52. Duo – much, many
53. Feng – maple
54. Guang – light
55. Hu – tiger
56. Ji – lucky
57. Kun – universe
58. Lin – forest
59. Mao – furry
60. Nuo – promise
61. Peizhi – respectful
62. Quan – fountain
63. Rui – sharp-minded
64. Shun – smooth, obedient
65. Ting – listen
66. Ushi – born at the time of the ox
67. Wen – culture, writing
68. Xiang – good luck
69. Yue – moon

70. Zian – self peace
71. Ai – love
72. Bin – refined
73. Chang – long
74. Dingxiang – stability and fortune
75. Er – ear
76. Fu – wealthy
77. Guan-yin – god of mercy
78. Heng – eternal
79. Jianyu – building the universe
80. Kuan-yin – buddhist deity of mercy
81. Liang – bright
82. Mao – fur, feathers
83. Nian – thinking
84. Peng – friend
85. Qilin – mythical creature
86. Ren – benevolence
87. Shu – warm-hearted
88. Tian – heaven
89. Uang – strength
90. Wei – towering
91. Xue – snow
92. Yaozu – respectful
93. Zian – self peace
94. An – peaceful
95. Bo – waves
96. Chen – morning
97. De – virtue
98. Fai – growth
99. Guo – country
100. Hui – intelligent

Hong Kong baby boy names

1. Aaron - Enlightened one
2. Adrian - Dark one
3. Alan - Handsome one
4. Alexander - Protector of mankind
5. Alfred - Wise counselor
6. Andrew - Manly, brave
7. Anthony - Priceless one
8. Austin - Majestic dignity
9. Benjamin - Son of the right hand
10. Brandon - Little raven
11. Brian - Noble, strong
12. Calvin - Bald
13. Charles - Free man
14. Chester - Fortress, walled town
15. Daniel - God is my judge
16. David - Beloved
17. Derek - People ruler
18. Donald - World ruler
19. Edward - Wealthy guardian
20. Ethan - Firm, strong
21. Felix - Happy, lucky
22. Francis - Free man
23. Gabriel - God is my strength
24. Gary - Spear rule
25. George - Farmer
26. Harold - Army ruler
27. Henry - Estate ruler
28. Howard - High guardian
29. Isaac - He will laugh
30. Jack - God is gracious
31. Jason - Healer
32. Jerry - Ruler with a spear
33. John - God is gracious

34. Joseph - He will add
35. Kevin - Handsome, beautiful
36. Larry - Laurel crowned
37. Leo - Lion
38. Louis - Famous warrior
39. Mark - Warlike
40. Michael - Who is like God?
41. Nathan - He gave
42. Neil - Champion
43. Oliver - Olive tree
44. Oscar - Friend of deer
45. Patrick - Nobleman
46. Peter - Rock
47. Ralph - Wolf counsel
48. Raymond - Wise protector
49. Richard - Brave power
50. Robert - Bright fame
51. Roger - Famous spear
52. Samuel - God has heard
53. Simon - He has heard
54. Stanley - Stony meadow
55. Stephen - Crown
56. Theodore - God's gift
57. Thomas - Twin
58. Timothy - Honoring God
59. Victor - Conqueror
60. Vincent - Conquering
61. Walter - Army ruler
62. William - Resolute protector
63. Winston - Joy stone
64. Zachary - God has remembered
65. Albert - Noble, bright
66. Arnold - Eagle power
67. Bernard - Brave as a bear
68. Bruce - From the brushwood thicket
69. Clifford - Ford by a cliff

70. Dennis - Follower of Dionysius
71. Edwin - Rich friend
72. Geoffrey - Peaceful ruler
73. Gilbert - Bright pledge
74. Herman - Army man
75. Leonard - Brave lion
76. Maurice - Dark-skinned
77. Norman - Northman
78. Oswald - God's power
79. Reginald - Advice ruler
80. Roland - Famous land
81. Sidney - Wide meadow
82. Terence - Tender, gracious
83. Wallace - Foreigner, stranger
84. Gerald - Ruler with a spear
85. Martin - Warlike
86. Alvin - Friend of elves
87. Erwin - Friend of the sea
88. Gordon - Large fortress
89. Melvin - Gentle lord
90. Orville - Golden city
91. Percival - Pierce the valley
92. Quentin - Fifth
93. Rupert - Bright fame
94. Sheldon - Steep valley
95. Todd - Fox
96. Wayne - Wagon maker
97. Xavier - New house
98. Yves - Yew wood
99. Zane - God is gracious
100. Nigel - Dark night

Macau baby boy names

1. Aiden – Fire
2. Aaron – High mountain
3. Adam – Man
4. Adrian – Rich
5. Alex – Defender
6. Andrew – Manly
7. Anthony – Priceless
8. Arthur – Noble
9. Ben – Son of the right hand
10. Benjamin – Son of the right hand
11. Bernard – Brave as a bear
12. Brian – High, noble
13. Calvin – Bald
14. Charles – Free man
15. Christian – Follower of Christ
16. Christopher – Christ-bearer
17. Daniel – God is my judge
18. David – Beloved
19. Derek – People's ruler
20. Dominic – Belonging to the Lord
21. Edward – Wealthy guardian
22. Ethan – Strong, firm
23. Felix – Happy, fortunate
24. Francis – Free man
25. Gabriel – God is my strength
26. George – Farmer
27. Harry – Home ruler
28. Henry – Ruler of the home
29. Isaac – He will laugh
30. Jack – God is gracious
31. Jacob – Supplanter
32. James – Supplanter
33. Jason – Healer

34. Jesse – Gift
35. John – God is gracious
36. Jonathan – God has given
37. Joseph – He will add
38. Joshua – The Lord is salvation
39. Justin – Just, fair
40. Kevin – Handsome, beautiful
41. Kyle – Narrow
42. Lawrence – From Laurentum
43. Leo – Lion
44. Liam – Helmet of will
45. Luke – Light giving
46. Mark – Warlike
47. Martin – Warlike
48. Matthew – Gift of God
49. Michael – Who is like God?
50. Nathan – He gave
51. Nicholas – Victory of the people
52. Noah – Rest, comfort
53. Oliver – Olive tree
54. Patrick – Nobleman
55. Paul – Small
56. Peter – Rock
57. Philip – Lover of horses
58. Ralph – Wolf counsel
59. Richard – Brave ruler
60. Robert – Bright fame
61. Roger – Famous spear
62. Samuel – God has heard
63. Sean – God is gracious
64. Simon – He has heard
65. Stephen – Crown
66. Thomas – Twin
67. Timothy – Honoring God
68. Victor – Conqueror
69. Vincent – Conquering

70. William – Resolute protector
71. Zachary – The Lord has remembered
72. Albert – Noble, bright
73. Arnold – Eagle power
74. Bruce – From the brushwood thicket
75. Chester – Fort
76. Clifford – Ford by a cliff
77. Dennis – Follower of Dionysius
78. Edmund – Wealthy protector
79. Ernest – Serious, determined
80. Geoffrey – Peaceful territory
81. Gilbert – Bright pledge
82. Howard – High guardian
83. Leonard – Brave lion
84. Maurice – Dark-skinned
85. Norman – Northman
86. Oswald – God's power
87. Percy – Pierce valley
88. Raymond – Wise protector
89. Reginald – Counsel power
90. Roland – Famous land
91. Sidney – Wide meadow
92. Stanley – Stony meadow
93. Terence – Tender, gracious
94. Wallace – Foreigner
95. Walter – Army ruler
96. Wilfred – Desiring peace
97. Xavier – New house
98. Yves – Yew wood
99. Zacharias – The Lord has remembered
100. Zephyr – West wind

Tibetan baby boy names

1. Tenzin - Protector of Dharma
2. Dorje - Indestructible
3. Wangchuk - Powerful
4. Norbu - Jewel
5. Sonam - Merit
6. Lobsang - Pure mind
7. Jigme - Fearless
8. Pema - Lotus
9. Thupten - Increase of teachings
10. Ngawang - Power of speech
11. Sherab - Wisdom
12. Kalsang - Good fortune
13. Rinchen - Precious gem
14. Karma - Action
15. Gyatso - Ocean
16. Tsultrim - Ethical discipline
17. Yonten - Wealth of knowledge
18. Chogyal - Dharma king
19. Chophel - Dharma flourishing
20. Trinley - Buddhist activity
21. Wangdue - Power to command
22. Chime - Immortal
23. Gyaltsen - Victory banner
24. Tashi - Good fortune
25. Dawa - Moon
26. Jamyang - Gentle voice
27. Tharchin - Stability
28. Sangey - Buddha
29. Palden - Glorious
30. Lhundup - Spontaneous
31. Tsewang - Life power
32. Drakpa - Brave
33. Gyalpo - King

34. Dechen - Great bliss
35. Tseten - Long life
36. Chokyi - Dharma joy
37. Tsedrup - Increase of life
38. Phuntsok - Excellent
39. Yeshe - Wisdom
40. Samten - Meditation
41. Gendun - Infinite joy
42. Tsering - Long life
43. Penpa - Benefactor
44. Yeshi - Wisdom
45. Rinzin - Holder of jewels
46. Thubten - Buddha's teachings
47. Choden - Religious
48. Drukpa - Dragon
49. Ngodup - Self accomplished
50. Jampa - Loving kindness
51. Thaye - Limitless
52. Lhawang - Divine power
53. Rabten - Steadfast
54. Nyima - Sun
55. Kunga - All joyous
56. Topden - Supreme
57. Dondrup - Fulfilled
58. Gyalwa - Victorious
59. Lhakpa - Wednesday
60. Chokden - Supreme dharma
61. Dakpa - Brave
62. Tashi - Auspicious
63. Jamtso - Gentle brother
64. Lhamo - Goddess
65. Kunchok - Rare and supreme
66. Lekdan - Fine wisdom
67. Tsegyal - Life victorious
68. Rigzin - Holder of knowledge
69. Chokphel - Dharma flourishing

70. Gyaltsen - Victory banner
71. Jigten - Worldly
72. Palden - Glorious
73. Thrinley - Buddhist activity
74. Tsewang - Life power
75. Dondrub - Accomplished
76. Ngawang - Mighty speech
77. Samphel - Spontaneous
78. Phurba - Dagger
79. Tenzing - Upholder of teachings
80. Tharpa - Liberation
81. Dhondup - Fulfilled wish
82. Gawa - Joy
83. Chime - Immortal
84. Dakpa - Brave
85. Rabsel - Clear light
86. Chogyam - Great dharma
87. Tashi - Lucky
88. Lobsang - Pure mind
89. Rigdol - Upholder of knowledge
90. Thokmay - Unobstructed
91. Khedup - Aspiration fulfilled
92. Delek - Happiness
93. Lhundrup - Spontaneous
94. Tashi - Fortune
95. Penjo - Dharma increasing
96. Wangyal - Power of charm
97. Chokden - Supreme dharma
98. Kelsang - Good fortune
99. Namgyal - Victorious in all directions
100. Kunchen - All knowing

Maldivian baby boy names

1. Aahil – Prince
2. Aariz – Respectable
3. Aayan – God's gift
4. Aadil – Just, Honest
5. Aafi – One who forgives
6. Aakif – Devoted
7. Aalam – World
8. Aamil – Doer
9. Aarif – Knowing, Aware
10. Aasim – One who restrains
11. Aayan – Gift of God
12. Abaan – Old Arabic name
13. Abbas – Lion
14. Abdul – Servant of God
15. Abid – Worshipper
16. Abir – Fragrance
17. Abrar – Piety
18. Adam – Man, Earth
19. Adil – Fair, Honest
20. Adnan – Settler
21. Afif – Chaste, Modest
22. Afiq – Honest
23. Afzal – Best, Superior
24. Ahad – One, Unique
25. Ahmad – Most praised
26. Ahmed – Most commendable
27. Ahsan – Perfection, Excellence
28. Aiman – Fearless
29. Aizat – Nobility
30. Ajmal – Most beautiful
31. Akbar – Great
32. Akif – Focused
33. Akram – Most generous

34. Alam – World, Universe
35. Ali – Exalted, Noble
36. Alim – Wise, Learned
37. Ameen – Faithful, Trustworthy
38. Amir – Prince, Leader
39. Amjad – More glorious
40. Anas – Affection, Love
41. Anis – Close friend
42. Anwar – Luminous
43. Aqil – Intelligent
44. Arif – Wise, Intelligent
45. Asad – Lion
46. Asif – Gather, Harvest
47. Asim – Protector
48. Atif – Compassionate, Affectionate
49. Ayaz – Cool Breeze
50. Ayman – Lucky, Blessed
51. Azhar – Shining, Bright
52. Azim – Determined
53. Aziz – Powerful, Beloved
54. Badr – Full moon
55. Bahir – Dazzling, Brilliant
56. Basim – Smiling
57. Bilal – Water, Moisture
58. Burhan – Proof
59. Daanish – Wisdom, Learning
60. Daud – Beloved
61. Faiz – Victorious
62. Faraz – Elevation
63. Farid – Unique
64. Faris – Horseman, Knight
65. Faisal – Decisive
66. Faiyaz – Artistic
67. Ghazi – Warrior
68. Habib – Beloved
69. Hafiz – Protector

70. Haidar – Lion
71. Hamid – Praiseworthy
72. Hamza – Lion
73. Haris – Guardian, Protector
74. Hasan – Handsome
75. Hashim – Destroyer of evil
76. Hussain – Handsome
77. Ibrahim – Father of multitude
78. Idris – Studious person
79. Ihsan – Beneficence
80. Imad – Support, Pillar
81. Imran – Prosperity
82. Irfan – Gratefulness
83. Isa – Jesus
84. Ismail – God will hear
85. Jamal – Beauty
86. Jawad – Generous
87. Jibril – Archangel Gabriel
88. Karim – Generous
89. Khalid – Eternal
90. Khurram – Delighted
91. Majid – Noble
92. Malik – King
93. Mubarak – Blessed
94. Mustafa – Chosen one
95. Nabeel – Noble
96. Naseer – Helper
97. Omar – Long-lived
98. Osman – Servant of God
99. Rafiq – Kind, Friend
100. Zahir – Bright, Shining

Mauritian baby boy names

1. Aarav - Peaceful
2. Abhinav - Innovative
3. Aditya - The Sun
4. Akash - Sky
5. Aman - Peace
6. Anish - Supreme
7. Ankit - Conquered
8. Arjun - Bright, shining
9. Ashish - Blessing
10. Avinash - Indestructible
11. Ayush - Long life
12. Bhavesh - Lord of the world
13. Chirag - Lamp
14. Darshan - Vision
15. Deepak - Light
16. Dhruv - Pole star
17. Eshan - Desiring and wishing
18. Gaurav - Pride
19. Harish - Lord Vishnu
20. Ishaan - Sun
21. Jai - Victory
22. Jayesh - Winner
23. Keshav - Another name for Lord Krishna
24. Kishan - Lord Krishna
25. Lakshman - Prosperous
26. Manish - God of mind
27. Mohan - Charming
28. Naveen - New
29. Omkar - Sound of Om
30. Prakash - Light
31. Rajesh - King
32. Rakesh - Lord of the night
33. Ravi - Sun

34. Rohit - Red
35. Sachin - Pure
36. Sameer - Wind
37. Sanjay - Triumphant
38. Suresh - Lord of Gods
39. Tarun - Young
40. Uday - Rising
41. Vimal - Pure
42. Yash - Glory
43. Abhay - Fearless
44. Amol - Priceless
45. Brijesh - Lord of Brij
46. Dinesh - Sun
47. Girish - Lord of mountains
48. Harsh - Happiness
49. Jagdish - Lord of the world
50. Kamal - Lotus
51. Lokesh - Lord of the world
52. Mahesh - Lord Shiva
53. Navin - New
54. Parth - Arjun
55. Pranav - Sacred syllable Om
56. Raman - Pleasing
57. Ritesh - Lord of truth
58. Sagar - Sea
59. Shyam - Dark
60. Sushil - Good character
61. Tushar - Snow
62. Vijay - Victory
63. Yuvraj - Prince
64. Ajay - Unconquered
65. Anurag - Love
66. Bimal - Pure
67. Devansh - Part of God
68. Gautam - Bright
69. Hitesh - Lord of goodness

70. Jeet - Victory
71. Kapil - Fair complexioned
72. Madhav - Sweet like honey
73. Nandan - Rejoicing
74. Pradeep - Light
75. Rajan - King
76. Roshan - Bright
77. Sharad - Autumn
78. Surya - Sun
79. Vijendra - Victorious
80. Yogesh - Lord of Yoga
81. Amit - Infinite
82. Ankur - Sprout
83. Chetan - Consciousness
84. Dheeraj - Patience
85. Gopal - Cowherd
86. Hemant - Winter
87. Jatin - Ascetic
88. Krish - Short form of Lord Krishna
89. Manoj - Born of the mind
90. Nikhil - Whole
91. Piyush - Milk
92. Rahul - Conqueror of miseries
93. Samar - War
94. Siddharth - One who has attained enlightenment
95. Trilok - Three worlds
96. Varun - Lord of water
97. Abhishek - Ritual
98. Anil - Wind
99. Brij - Place of Lord Krishna
100. Chandan - Sandalwood

Seychellois baby boy names

1. Aaron - Enlightened
2. Abel - Breath
3. Abraham - Father of many
4. Adam - Man
5. Adrian - From Hadria
6. Aiden - Little fire
7. Alan - Handsome
8. Albert - Noble and bright
9. Alexander - Defender of the people
10. Alfred - Wise counselor
11. Andrew - Manly
12. Anthony - Priceless one
13. Arthur - Bear
14. Austin - Majestic
15. Benjamin - Son of the right hand
16. Bernard - Brave as a bear
17. Brandon - From the broom hill
18. Brian - High or noble
19. Bruce - From the brushwood thicket
20. Caleb - Faithful
21. Calvin - Bald
22. Carl - Free man
23. Charles - Free man
24. Christian - Follower of Christ
25. Christopher - Bearer of Christ
26. Daniel - God is my judge
27. David - Beloved
28. Dennis - Devotee of Dionysus
29. Derek - People's ruler
30. Dominic - Belonging to the Lord
31. Donald - World ruler
32. Douglas - Dark stream
33. Dylan - Son of the sea

34. Edward - Wealthy guardian
35. Elijah - The Lord is my God
36. Eric - Eternal ruler
37. Ethan - Firm, enduring
38. Eugene - Well-born
39. Evan - God is gracious
40. Felix - Happy, fortunate
41. Francis - Free man
42. Frank - Free man
43. Gabriel - God is my strength
44. Gary - Spearman
45. George - Farmer
46. Gerald - Ruler with the spear
47. Gilbert - Bright pledge
48. Gordon - Large fortification
49. Graham - Gravelly homestead
50. Gregory - Watchful, alert
51. Harold - Army ruler
52. Harry - Army ruler
53. Henry - Ruler of the home
54. Howard - High guardian
55. Hugh - Mind, intellect
56. Ian - God is gracious
57. Isaac - He will laugh
58. Jack - God is gracious
59. Jacob - Supplanter
60. James - Supplanter
61. Jason - Healer
62. Jeffrey - Peaceful traveler
63. Jeremy - God will uplift
64. Jesse - Gift
65. Joel - Yahweh is God
66. John - God is gracious
67. Joseph - He will add
68. Joshua - The Lord is my salvation
69. Julian - Youthful

70. Justin - Just, fair
71. Keith - Wood
72. Kenneth - Handsome
73. Kevin - Kind, gentle
74. Kyle - Narrow
75. Lawrence - From Laurentum
76. Leonard - Brave as a lion
77. Leroy - The king
78. Lewis - Renowned warrior
79. Logan - Small hollow
80. Louis - Renowned warrior
81. Lucas - Light
82. Luke - Light
83. Mark - Warlike
84. Martin - Warlike
85. Matthew - Gift of God
86. Michael - Who is like God?
87. Nathan - He gave
88. Nathaniel - Gift of God
89. Neil - Champion
90. Nicholas - People's victory
91. Oliver - Olive tree
92. Oscar - Friend of deer
93. Patrick - Nobleman
94. Paul - Small
95. Peter - Rock
96. Philip - Lover of horses
97. Ralph - Wolf counsel
98. Raymond - Wise protector
99. Richard - Brave ruler
100. Robert - Bright fame

nt English Baby Boy Names

- Fire
Alden - Old friend
Alvin - Noble friend
Ansel - God's protection
Arden - Eagle valley
Baldwin - Bold friend
Barrett - Bear strength
Beckett - Bee cottage
Bede - Prayer
Bertram - Bright raven
Cedric - Bounty
Cuthbert - Famous brilliant
Eadric - Wealthy ruler
Edgar - Wealthy spearman
Edwin - Wealthy friend
Egbert - Bright edge
Elwin - Elf friend
Erwin - Sea friend
Ethelbert - Noble and bright
Everett - Wild boar herd
Farnham - Fern field
Godric - God's ruler
Harold - Army power
Harlan - Rocky land
Heath - Wasteland
Hedley - Heather meadow
Leofric - Beloved ruler
Leopold - Bold people
Linus - Flaxen
Mervyn - Sea hill

Osbert - Divine bright
Oswald - Divine power
Percival - Pierce the valley
Radcliffe - Red cliff
Redmond - Wise protector
Reginald - Advice ruler
Roderick - Famous power
Roland - Famous land
Rupert - Bright fame
Selwyn - Friend in the castle
Stanley - Stony meadow
Thurstan - Thor's stone
Ulfred - Wolf peace
Wilfred - Desires peace
Wystan - Battle stone
Yorick - Farmer
Alaric - Ruler of all people
Godwin - God's friend
Eamon - Rich protector
Ivor - Archer's bow.

Royal Baby Boy Names

Albert - Noble and bright
Alfred - Wise counselor
Arthur - Bear, strong as a bear
Alexander - Defender of men
Andrew - Manly, brave
Benedict - Blessed
Charles - Free man
Christian - Follower of Christ
David - Beloved
Edward - Wealthy guardian
Frederick - Peaceful ruler
George - Farmer
Harold - Army ruler
Henry - Ruler of the home
James - Supplanter
John - God is gracious
Louis - Famous warrior
Michael - Who is like God?
Nicholas - Victory of the people
Oliver - Olive tree
Philip - Lover of horses
Richard - Powerful ruler
Robert - Bright fame
Stephen - Crown
William - Resolute protector
Victor - Conqueror
Thomas - Twin
Samuel - Heard by God
Peter - Rock
Paul - Small

Oscar - Friend of deer
Maximilian - Greatest
Leopold - Bold people
Julian - Youthful, downy
Hugh - Mind, intellect
Gregory - Watchful, alert
Geoffrey - Peaceful territory
Francis - Free man
Ernest - Serious, resolute
Edmund - Wealthy protector
Dominic - Belonging to the Lord
Daniel - God is my judge
Christopher - Bearer of Christ
Benjamin - Son of the right hand
Anthony - Priceless one
Adrian - From Hadria
Aaron - High mountain
Gabriel - God is my strength
Raphael - God has healed
Zachary - The Lord has remembered

Literary Baby Boy Names

Atticus - From Harper Lee's "To Kill a Mockingbird," means "man of Attica."

Holden - From J.D. Salinger's "The Catcher in the Rye," means "deep valley."

Gatsby - From F. Scott Fitzgerald's "The Great Gatsby," means "left-handed."

Dorian - From Oscar Wilde's "The Picture of Dorian Gray," means "child of the sea."

Heathcliff - From Emily Bronte's "Wuthering Heights," means "cliff near a heath."

Rhett - From Margaret Mitchell's "Gone with the Wind," means "advice."

Jay - From "The Great Gatsby," means "jaybird."

Sawyer - From Mark Twain's "Tom Sawyer," means "wood cutter."

Romeo - From Shakespeare's "Romeo and Juliet," means "pilgrim to Rome."

Darcy - From Jane Austen's "Pride and Prejudice," means "dark one."

Huckleberry - From Mark Twain's "Huckleberry Finn," means "sweet berry."

Pip - From Charles Dickens' "Great Expectations," means "lover of horses."

Oliver - From Charles Dickens' "Oliver Twist," means "olive tree."

Edgar - From Edgar Allan Poe, means "wealthy spearman."

Oscar - From Oscar Wilde, means "God spear."

Ernest - From Oscar Wilde's "The Importance of Being Earnest," means "serious."

Algernon - From Oscar Wilde's "The Importance of Being Earnest," means "with a moustache."

Jem - From Harper Lee's "To Kill a Mockingbird," means "supplanter."

Hamlet - From Shakespeare's "Hamlet," means "little home."

Othello - From Shakespeare's "Othello," means "wealthy."

Sherlock - From Arthur Conan Doyle's "Sherlock Holmes," means "bright hair."

Marcel - From Marcel Proust, means "little warrior."

Finn - From Mark Twain's "Huckleberry Finn," means "fair."

George - From John Steinbeck's "Of Mice and Men," means "farmer."

Nick - From "The Great Gatsby," means "victory of the people."

Scout - From Harper Lee's "To Kill a Mockingbird," means "to listen."

Quentin - From William Faulkner's "The Sound and the Fury," means "fifth."

Ahab - From Herman Melville's "Moby Dick," means "uncle."

Ishmael - Also from "Moby Dick," means "God will hear."

Lennie - From John Steinbeck's "Of Mice and Men," means "lion strength."

Silas - From George Eliot's "Silas Marner," means "wood, forest."

Tristan - From Thomas Hardy's "Tristram of Lyonesse," means "tumult, outcry."

Arthur - From Arthur Conan Doyle, means "bear."

Beowulf - From "Beowulf," means "bee wolf."

Frodo - From J.R.R. Tolkien's "Lord of the Rings," means "wise by experience."

Sam - Also from "Lord of the Rings," means "told by God."

Aragorn - Also from "Lord of the Rings," means "revered king."

Bilbo - From J.R.R. Tolkien's "The Hobbit," means "sword."

Gulliver - From Jonathan Swift's "Gulliver's Travels," means "glutton."

Hester - From Nathaniel Hawthorne's "The Scarlet Letter," means "star."

Tom - From Mark Twain's "Tom Sawyer," means "twin."

Samsa - From Franz Kafka's "The Metamorphosis," means "being alone."

Gregor - Also from "The Metamorphosis," means "watchful, alert."

Ivan - From Fyodor Dostoevsky's "The Brothers Karamazov," means "God is gracious."

Alex - From Anthony Burgess' "A Clockwork Orange," means "defender of men."

Humbert - From Vladimir Nabokov's "Lolita," means "bright warrior."

Raskolnikov - From Fyodor Dostoevsky's "Crime and Punishment," means "split."

Winston - From George Orwell's "1984," means "joy stone."

Isherwood - From Christopher Isherwood, means "iron wood."

Melville - From Herman Melville, means "bad settlement."

Native American Baby Boy Names

Ahote - Restless one
Akecheta - Fighter
Bidziil - He is strong
Chayton - Falcon
Cheveyo - Spirit warrior
Delsin - He is so
Elsu - Flying falcon
Enapay - Brave
Etu - Sun
Eyota - Great
Hakan - Fire
Haloke - Salmon
Hok'ee - Abandoned
Honi - Wolf
Hotah - White
Hototo - Warrior spirit who sings
Howi - Turtle dove
Huritt - Handsome
Kachada - White man
Kangee - Raven
Kitchi - Brave
Kohana - Swift
Koko - Night
Len - Flute
Mato - Bear
Micco - Chief
Niyol - Wind
Nodin - Wind
Ohanzee - Shadow
Onacona - White owl

Osyka - Eagle
Pachu'a - Feathered water snake
Peta - Golden eagle
Qaletaqa - Guardian of the people
Sahale - Above
Sik'is - Friend
Sunki - To catch up with
Tadi - Wind
Takoda - Friend to everyone
Tse - Rock
Viho - Chief
Wakiza - Desperate warrior
Wematin - Brother
Wicasa - Sage
Wikvaya - One who brings
Wiyaka - Feather
Yuma - Son of the chief
Zihna - Spins
Ahanu - He laughs
Chankoowashtay - Good road.

Aboriginal Baby Boy Names

Apari - Means "father" in Australian Aboriginal language.

Bardo - Means "water" in Australian Aboriginal language.

Coen - A name of a town in Queensland, Australia.

Daku - Means "sand hill" in Australian Aboriginal language.

Erro - Means "sun" in Australian Aboriginal language.

Jiemba - Means "laughing star" in Wiradjuri language.

Koa - Means "crow" in Australian Aboriginal language.

Lurnea - Means "a resting place" in Aboriginal language.

Miro - A type of tree in Australia.

Naretha - Means "blue water" in Australian Aboriginal language.

Omeo - A name of a town in Victoria, Australia.

Pindan - Means "red earth" in Australian Aboriginal language.

Quoba - Means "snake" in Australian Aboriginal language.

Taree - A name of a town in New South Wales, Australia.

Ulo - Means "owl" in Australian Aboriginal language.

Warrigal - Means "wild" in Australian Aboriginal language.

Yarran - A type of tree in Australia.

Zarek - Means "sunrise" in Australian Aboriginal language.

Jarli - Means "barn owl" in Australian Aboriginal language.

Kuparr - Means "red earth" in Australian Aboriginal language.

Lowan - Means "mallee fowl" in Australian Aboriginal language.

Marlu - Means "kangaroo" in Australian Aboriginal language.

Nyungar - Means "people" in Australian Aboriginal language.

Orana - Means "welcome" in Australian Aboriginal language.

Parri - Means "river" in Australian Aboriginal language.

Quilpie - A name of a town in Queensland, Australia.

Tarka - Means "eggshell" in Australian Aboriginal language.

Uluru - A famous rock formation in Australia.

Warrin - Means "winter" in Australian Aboriginal language.

Yaraan - A type of tree in Australia.

Zephyr - Means "west wind" in Australian Aboriginal language.

Jardi - Means "sea" in Australian Aboriginal language.

Kupala - Means "fire" in Australian Aboriginal language.

Lue - A name of a town in New South Wales, Australia.

Mungo - A name of a national park in Australia.

Narran - A name of a lake in Australia.

Oratunga - A name of a creek in Australia.

Parramatta - A suburb in Sydney, Australia.

Quandong - A type of fruit in Australia.

Tumut - A name of a town in New South Wales, Australia.

Ulan - A name of a town in New South Wales, Australia.

Wollomombi - A name of a waterfall in Australia.

Yarramundi - An influential Aboriginal man in the early days of British settlement.

Zanthus - A name of a town in Western Australia.

Jarrah - A type of tree in Australia.

Kari - Means "fire" in Australian Aboriginal language.

Leumeah - Means "here I rest" in Australian Aboriginal language.

Mungana - A name of a town in Queensland, Australia.

Nymboida - A name of a river in New South Wales, Australia.

Oodnadatta - A name of a town in South Australia.

Maroi Baby Boy Names

Aroha -   "love"
Tane -   "man"
Mana -   "authority, power"
Rangi -   "sky"
Ihaia -   "God is salvation"
Kauri - Named after a large native tree in New Zealand
Tamati -   "twin"
Hemi -   "home ruler"
Wiremu -   "resolute protector"
Tama -   "son, boy"
Rongo -   "peace"
Hori -   "farmer"
Matiu -   "gift of God"
Kahurangi -   "treasured possession"
Tai -   "tide"
Whetu -   "star"
Ariki -   "chief"
Hoani -   "God is gracious"
Kahu -   "harrier hawk"
Nikau - Named after a native palm tree in New Zealand
Rawiri -   "beloved"
Tawhiri -   "wind"
Hare -   "happy"
Raukura -   "red feather"
Tuhoe - Named after a Maori tribe
Whero -   "red"
Taika -   "tiger"
Piri -   "close, join"

Manawa - "heart, mind"
Turoa - "long standing"
Tangaroa - "god of the sea"
Tama-nui-te-ra - "great sun"
Te Ariki - "the lord"
Rata - Named after a native tree in New Zealand
Te Rangi - "the day"
Mikaere - "who is like God"
Te Mana - "the authority"
Te Kahu - "the cloak"
Te Whetu - "the star"
Te Hau - "the wind"
Te Aroha - "the love"
Te Moana - "the sea"
Te Rau - "the leaf"
Te Ao - "the world"
Te Tai - "the tide"
Te Wai - "the water"
Te Marama - "the moon"
Te Rua - "the pit, grave"
Te Hiku - "the tail"
Te One - "the sand"

Sami Baby Boy Names

Ailu - Wealthy
Aki - Noble
Ante - Beyond praise
Aslak - God-like
Biret - The exalted one
Eino - Lone warrior
Elle - Light
Esa - God is my salvation
Gaute - Goth, Gaut
Haldor - Rock of Thor
Heiki - Home ruler
Iisakki - He will laugh
Jalmari - Helmeted warrior
Jari - Helmeted warrior
Jouni - God is gracious
Juhani - God is gracious
Kaarlo - Free man
Kari - Pure
Kustaa - Staff of the gods
Lasse - Crowned with laurels
Leif - Heir, descendant
Mauno - Great
Niilo - Champion
Oiva - Excellent
Paavo - Small
Pertti - Noble, bright
Pekka - Rock
Rauno - Counsel, advice
Risto - Christ-bearer
Sakari - God remembers

Seppo - Smith
Taavi - Beloved
Tapio - God of the forest
Toivo - Hope
Turo - Thor's bear
Ukko - Old man
Valtteri - Ruler of the army
Väinö - Wide, broad
Yrjö - Farmer
Aatu - Noble wolf
Eemeli - Rival
Ilmari - Air
Jorma - Farmer
Kalle - Free man
Lauri - Laurel
Martti - Warlike
Niko - Victory of the people
Onni - Happiness, luck
Riku - Rich, powerful ruler
Sampo - Magical artifact.

Inuit Baby Boy Names

Akiak - Brave
Nanook - Polar Bear
Kavik - Wolverine
Miki - Little
Suka - Fast
Tukkuttok - Hard Stone
Akna - Mother Goddess
Nukilik - Strong
Pana - God of Hunting
Sakari - Sweet
Atiqtalik - Polar Bear Mother
Panik - Daughter
Kallik - Lightning
Sesi - Snow
Koko - Chocolate
Mauja - Soft Deep Snow
Aput - Snow
Siku - Ice
Qimmiq - Dog
Ivik - Base of a cliff
Pukiq - Smart
Tootega - Man of Sea
Kunik - Kiss
Oki - Man
Sura - New Life
Tukkuttog - Flint
Uki - Survivor
Ila - Friend
Inuk - Person
Kaskae - Chief

Nanuq - Polar Bear
Qaletaqa - Guardian of People
Siku - Sea Ice
Tootega - Man of Sea
Uki - Survivor
Yuralria - Dancer
Amaqjuaq - The Strong One
Ijiraq - Shape Shifter
Qimugjuk - Husky Dog
Taktu - Harpoon
Ubluriak - Wolf
Yuka - Bright Stars
Anirniq - Breath
Iqniq - Fire
Qajaq - Kayak
Tupit - Tattoos
Ukiuk - Winter
Yuralria - Dancer
Anana - Beautiful
Ivalu - Sinew.

Hawiian Baby Boy Names

Akamu - Form of Adam, "earth"
Keanu - Means "the cool breeze" in Hawaiian
Palani - Free man or from France
Meka - Eyes
Kekoa - The brave one
Makani - Wind
Ikaika - Strong
Koa - Brave, fearless
Keoki - Form of George, "farmer"
Kaleo - The voice
Lono - God of peace and prosperity
Kealii - Chief
Kaimana - Power of the sea
Kahuna - Priest
Mano - Shark
Kalani - The heavens
Kapono - The good one
Kailani - Sea and sky
Keani - The wave, or breeze over the water
Nohea - Lovely
Alika - Most beautiful
Mael - Chief or prince
Keahi - Flames
Makoa - Fearless
Kainoa - Free-flowing ocean
Hani - Happy, joy
Kekipi - The rebel
Akela - Wisdom
Keola - Life
Kanoa - The free one

Kaili - God
Nui - Important
Kala - Sun
Manu - Bird
Kaipo - Sweetheart
Pika - Rock
Kolohe - Little rascal
Pekelo - Stone
Liko - Bud
Kealoha - Love
Iolana - To soar like a hawk
Kahale - House
Kaimi - The seeker
Lahela - Innocent lamb
Lokela - Famous warrior
Pomaika'i - Lucky
Ka'aukai - Seafarer
Keawe - The twisted, the firm
Kupono - Righteous
Aouli - Blue sky.

Slavic Baby Boy Names

Aleksandr - Defender of mankind
Boris - Fighter
Casimir - Proclaims peace
Dragan - Precious
Evgeni - Noble
Fyodor - God's gift
Gavril - God is my strength
Havel - Little rock
Igor - Warrior of peace
Jarek - Spring
Karel - Free man
Lubomir - Peace and love
Miroslav - Peace and glory
Nenad - Unexpected
Oleg - Holy
Piotr - Rock, stone
Radomir - Happy peace
Stanislav - Glory and fame
Tihomir - Quiet peace
Uros - Lord
Vasil - Royal, kingly
Yaroslav - Bright glory
Zoran - Daylight
Dobry - Good
Branislav - Protector and glory
Vladimir - Ruler of the world
Svetozar - World of light
Dusan - Soul, spirit
Vojtech - Consoling soldier
Radovan - Happy joy

Lev - Lion
Milos - Lover of glory
Rostislav - Increase glory
Slavik - Glory
Vlado - Rule
Yegor - Farmer
Zbigniew - To dispel anger
Kazimir - Destroyer of peace
Leszek - Holly
Maksim - Greatest
Nikita - Unconquered
Oskar - Deer lover
Pavel - Small
Radek - Happy
Simeon - One who hears
Tomislav - Twin glory
Venceslav - More glory
Wojciech - Soldier's consolation
Yaromir - Peaceful spring
Zdenek - The one from Sidon

Saxon Baby Boy Names

Alden – Wise Friend
Alston – From the Elf's Home
Aric – Ruler of All
Baldwin – Brave Friend
Barrett – Mighty as a Bear
Bentley – Meadow with Coarse Grass
Beorn – Warrior
Brantley – Fire Brand
Colby – Coal Village
Deacon – Dusty One
Draven – Hunter
Edgar – Rich, Powerful
Edwin – Prosperous Friend
Elton – Ella's Town
Emerson – Son of Emery
Everley – Boar Meadow
Farley – Fern Wood
Garret – Spear Rule
Godric – God Ruler
Harold – Army Ruler
Harvey – Battle Worthy
Irwin – Sea Friend
Jagger – Carter
Keaton – Where Hawks Fly
Kelvin – River Man
Kenway – Brave Royal Fighter
Leighton – Leek Town
Lincoln – Lake Colony
Marlow – Drained Lake
Norton – North Town

Orson – Bear Cub
Osmond – God's Protection
Prescott – Priest's Cottage
Quentin – Fifth
Radley – Red Meadow
Ramsey – Garlic Island
Sheldon – Steep Valley
Sherwin – Bright Friend
Stanley – Stony Meadow
Sutton – South Town
Tennyson – Son of Dennis
Thane – Landowner
Triston – Tumult
Upton – High Town
Vance – Thresher
Wayland – Land by the Road
Wilfred – Desiring Peace
Xander – Defender of the People
York – Yew Tree Estate
Zane – God is Gracious

Nature Based Baby Boy Names

River - A large natural stream of water flowing in a channel to the sea, a lake, or another such stream.

Forest - A large area covered chiefly with trees and undergrowth.

Reed - A tall, slender-leaved plant of the grass family that grows in water or on marshy ground.

Rowan - A mountain ash tree, associated with wisdom and protection.

Flint - A hard type of rock, symbolizing strength.

Jasper - A precious stone, symbolizing treasure or valuable.

Orion - A prominent constellation, named after a hunter in Greek mythology.

Ash - A type of tree, symbolizing strength and endurance.

Blaze - A very large or fiercely burning fire, symbolizing passion and spirit.

Cliff - A high, steep face of rock or earth, symbolizing strength and stability.

Dale - A valley, symbolizing tranquility and peace.

Hawk - A bird of prey, symbolizing power and freedom.

Glen - A narrow valley, symbolizing peace and solitude.

Heath - A tract of open uncultivated land, symbolizing simplicity and openness.

Jay - A type of bird, symbolizing joy and happiness.

Linden - A type of tree, symbolizing protection and love.

Moss - A small flowerless green plant, symbolizing comfort and peace.

Oak - A type of tree, symbolizing strength and endurance.

Rain - Water falling from the sky, symbolizing life and renewal.

Sage - A type of herb, symbolizing wisdom and immortality.

Thorn - A sharp pointed spine or prickle, symbolizing defense and protection.

Vale - A valley, symbolizing peace and tranquility.

West - One of the four cardinal directions, symbolizing exploration and adventure.

Yarrow - A type of flowering plant, symbolizing healing and protection.

Zephyr - A soft gentle breeze, symbolizing freedom and lightness.

Birch - A type of tree, symbolizing new beginnings and cleansing of the past.

Cedar - A type of tree, symbolizing strength and healing.

Drake - A male duck, symbolizing resourcefulness and adaptability.

Elm - A type of tree, symbolizing dignity and grace.

Falcon - A bird of prey, symbolizing power and agility.

Grove - A small wood, symbolizing peace and tranquility.

Heron - A large fish-eating wading bird, symbolizing patience and long life.

Ivy - A type of climbing plant, symbolizing fidelity and eternity.

Kestrel - A small falcon, symbolizing speed and grace.

Lark - A songbird, symbolizing happiness and creativity.

Maple - A type of tree, symbolizing balance and promise.

North - One of the four cardinal directions, symbolizing wisdom and introspection.

Pine - A type of tree, symbolizing immortality and wisdom.

Quill - A main flight feather of a bird, symbolizing lightness and writing.

Ridge - A long narrow hilltop, symbolizing strength and stability.

Sparrow - A small bird, symbolizing joy and protection.

Tern - A seabird, symbolizing freedom and grace.

Upland - An area of high or hilly land, symbolizing strength and stability.

Vale - A valley, symbolizing peace and tranquility.

Wolf - A wild carnivorous mammal, symbolizing loyalty and spirit.

Yew - A type of tree, symbolizing death and resurrection.

Alder - A type of tree, symbolizing strength and resilience.

Brook - A small stream, symbolizing peace and tranquility.

Crane - A large, tall bird, symbolizing longevity and happiness.

Dune - A hill of sand built by the wind, symbolizing change and adaptability.

Ancient Irish Baby Boy Names

Aedan – Born of fire
Aidan – Little fiery one
Barra – Fair-haired
Beacan – Tiny one
Brady – Spirited, Broad
Brendan – Prince
Brian – High, noble
Caelan – Powerful warrior
Cathal – Strong in battle
Cian – Ancient, distant
Conan – Little wolf
Conall – Strong wolf
Cormac – Charioteer
Daire – Fertile, fruitful
Declan – Man of prayer
Dermot – Free man
Donnacha – Brown-haired warrior
Eamon – Guardian of the riches
Eoghan – Born of the yew tree
Fergus – Man of vigor
Finn – Fair
Fionn – Fair or white
Flann – Red, ruddy
Gallagher – Eager helper
Garbhan – Rough
Hugh – Mind, intellect
Keegan – Little fiery one
Kieran – Dark-haired
Lorcan – Little fierce one
Malachy – My messenger

Niall – Champion
Oisin – Little deer
Padraig – Nobleman
Quinlan – Very fit
Rian – Little king
Rory – Red king
Sean – God is gracious
Shane – God's gracious gift
Tadhg – Poet or philosopher
Tiernan – Little lord
Torin – Chief
Ultan – Man from Ulster
Vaughan – Little
Ruairi – Red king
Seamus – Supplanter
Darragh – Oak tree
Colm – Dove
Ciaran – Dark
Fiachra – Raven
Diarmuid – Without enemy

Printed in Dunstable, United Kingdom